I am taken by the way she recounts her journey… laughter amidst sorrow, joy interweaves with sorrow… then when hope ascends, I realize that Thiel's story is my own.

Hans Peterson
Masters of Theology and the Arts, Professional singer/songwriter

"Bitter and Sweet" is profound and full of feelings that come and go with loss, transition, grief, and love. Interspersed with humor and frustration, fun and sadness… all the opposites that happen during this kind of journey. Darcy is excellent at explaining reality, facing it while doing something about it! I felt as if I'm in a circle of friends she has asked to gather around her to listen deeply. She expresses worries that most people think about and feel but don't express unless they are in therapy!

Bonnie Collins, LCSW-R, Family Therapist

I highly recommend "Bitter and Sweet." It is more than just a book about critical illness, it is a book of love. The amazing love of a couple through sickness and health, the love of family and friends, God's love, and the love of a community. To witness this is life changing. It will inspire you to love those you care about more completely every day.

Janet Carr, Independent Book Proofer

Bitter and Sweet:
A Family's Journey with Cancer

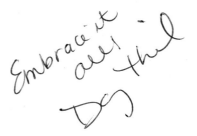

By Darcy Thiel MA, LMHC

Baby Coop Publishing, LLC

Publishing Coordinator: Karen Sharp-Price
Graphic Artist: Mark Krawczyk
Photos: Amber Coakley, Kristy Weiss
Permission: Diane Eble
Lyrics: Hans Peterson

ISBN: 978-0-9886101-0-1
Library of Congress Control Number: 2013900103

marriageandfamilycounseling.net
Baby Coop Publishing, LLC   West Seneca, NY
babycooppublishing.com

Manufactured in the United States of America

For Tim.

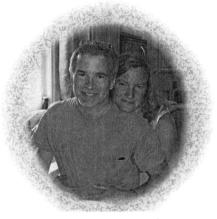

We did it, baby!

CONTENTS

ACKNOWLEDGEMENTS

This is a very difficult task for me, as I feel like in all honesty, there could be another book written just to mention all the people that have supported me and my family over the last few years. My worst fear is that I may forget to mention someone when so many have come to my aid. First, there are those people and entities that helped me/us get through our trauma, and still are here today as the journey never really ends. Those names I have tried to mention in the Introduction.

Then there is the arduous task of writing a book, which I have discovered involves a whole other army of people in order to do it well. First, I'd like to thank Amber Coakley from Birder's Lounge, and Kristy Weiss for use of their photographs. Thanks to Mark Krawczyk for his beautiful artwork on the cover, as well as his design layout for the book. I knew you could do it!

For all those accounting questions, many thanks to Kevin Gibson and Jan Piper for taking my countless calls with good humor.

Thanks to Hans Peterson, for not only writing the poignant words to "Everything is Grace", but also for graciously allowing us to use the lyrics. Thanks to the many editors that sacrificed their time and energy: Karen Sharp-Price, Janet Carr, Mark Krawczyk, Colleen McCoy, Teresa Sharp... I'm grateful to each of you!

To Chris, for the last 12 years of counseling, and Shirley for the last two years of spiritual direction, you are the places where I get centered. You are my "steadies," my sanity. My perspective. Thank you both.

Thanks to all the Hospice folks, especially Dr. Chris Kerr, Sue Herold and Rose Collins for going out of their way to help make this book a success.

What would I do without my Ya Ya's? You know who you are. Ever since my mother passed in 2007, I grow more aware every day that it is the women in your life that love you like no other. That is putting it mildly.

For being a prophetess, using all of your spiritual gifts with your usual whole hearted care and effort, for being the dearest friend ever, and for writing the Foreword for the book, I love you, Linda "B" Babcock.

I want to thank my family, who is my rock and foundation. The older I get, the more I realize how incredibly lucky I was to have grown up and lived my life with the family I've been surrounded with. They are here, through thick and thin. Through the beautiful and the ugly. Through the bitter and the sweet.

Without my son Timmy, I'm not sure what would have happened to Dave and me. Thank you for all the things you do every day. You do the cooking, cleaning, mowing, shoveling, child care, and most of all, you are Dave's best friend and favorite person in the world. Thanks for all those times you cleaned up my messes because I just couldn't get out of bed or function that day. And to the rest of my kids and grandkids - you are why I get up every day!

To Sallie Randolph, my publishing lawyer, my deepest thanks. So many endless phone calls, emails, questions and questions and questions. Your expertise was essential.

Karen Sharp-Price. There is no human way to possibly acknowledge what you have meant to me and this project. For months and months your endurance was greater than mine. You worked longer hours than I and patiently endured all my temper tantrums and attempts to give up. There were many work days where I was overcome with grief and you just hugged me and never budged. You are brilliant, dear friend. You are gifted, talented, and intelligent. There is no salary that could pay you your worth. I pray that somehow you will be blessed in the ways that you have blessed me and so many, many others. You're incredible!

Darcy Thiel

FOREWORD

"Bitter and Sweet" is a remarkable story of a woman and her family as they faced cancer and the subsequent death of a husband, father and grandfather. It was a privilege to walk the road with Darcy as she valiantly led Tim and his children from the initial terminal diagnosis to Tim's death in just five short months.

I first met Darcy and Tim when they joined the church and later Darcy and I became colleagues in ministry. We spent many hours together and subsequently forged a strong friendship built on common faith, shared trust, and a large measure of love and laughter. The running joke among the men in our lives was how much time we spent talking on the phone to one another. As it turned out, this phone connection would play a huge part in the way Darcy and I communicated during that chaotic time in her life. *Bitter* was the call I received while waiting for my daughter to walk the stage to receive her diploma from the out of state university she attended, as Darcy struggled to tell me through gulping sobs that Tim's routine gallbladder surgery had fast become a nightmare. The doctor had a high level suspicion that Tim had stage IV gallbladder cancer and he could not operate. That call was the first of hundreds over the course of the next five months. Some calls prompted immediate visits to the house or Hospice while others were to simply listen to Darcy as she grieved the husband and life that she knew was rapidly disappearing. *Sweet* were the late night calls when Tim and Darcy put the phone on the pillow between the two of them and the three of us would talk into the night trying to chase away the fear and darkness that loomed ahead.

The CaringBridge journal that Tim and Darcy created took on a life of its own as the two of them candidly shared the unknown path ahead of their family. The journal entries became a tangible way for family, friends, and co-workers, both near and far away, to share the family's suffering and offer prayers and support. Initially, Tim set his mind on "living strong" which he articulated in early journal entries. Once it became clear that living was not going to be an option, Tim set his mind on "dying strong." It is often said that dying takes a lot of energy and as a witness to Tim's death I can say that seems to be a true statement. Watching someone die takes perhaps even more energy and I witnessed Darcy take on that challenge with focused determination and courage that still leaves me filled with respect and awe.

Family and friends encouraged Darcy and Tim to have a benefit to help cover some of the expenses that would occur after Tim's untimely death, especially as they were raising an eight year old son. The family was overwhelmed by the response for help, donations and attendance and as the night of the benefit wore on Tim became too tired to stay to the end. I remember sitting in their living room with Tim as he rested and every now and again he would begin a conversation about something either totally on point or completely off topic and we would laugh. To this day when I see the movie "Overboard" on the TV menu I always watch it in tribute to Tim. Through some tears and with a smile on my face I recall our conversation wondering how people can fail to recognize that Kate Hudson is Goldie Hawn's daughter!

"Bitter and Sweet" will speak to the hearts of anyone who has suffered the loss of someone they held dear. It will be like a balm to wounded hearts and will resonate with those who despair about never getting beyond their pain and grief. More than anything else though, *"Bitter and Sweet"* is filled with tangible hope. It is one family's story of transformation from who they thought they were to who they subsequently became. Spanning every human emotion that cancer raises, readers may well find themselves crying, yelling and cheering as the Thiel-Colvin family alternately failed and succeeded along the way. Darcy writes with the same passion that she poured into caring for Tim during his last days and readers will surely be able to identify with any one of the people chronicled in her story. *Bitter* was the journey and *sweet* are the memories and I will forever be grateful and honored to have been one of the characters in this beautifully poignant story.

Linda Babcock
Director of Education and Mission,
Orchard Park Presbyterian Church

A Review of *Bitter and Sweet: A Family's Journey with Cancer*
Yuman Fong, MD
Professor of Surgery,
Memorial Sloan-Kettering Cancer Center

Cancer turns a patient's world upside down. In one moment, time goes from being counted forward from birth, to being counted backwards from death. A young 48 year old patient awaiting the weddings of his children and birth of grandchildren is suddenly 160 days from death. This is the frightful experience faced by 1.7 million Americans diagnosed with cancer yearly. Life immediately assumes a great urgency and uncertainty. That is why we grasp on to the inspirational stories of other cancer victims. We cherish the story of Chuck Pagano, the Indianapolis Colts football coach and we cried as we read the inspirational "The Last Lecture" about the courage with which Professor Randy Pausch fought and ultimately lost his fight against pancreatic cancer.

"Bitter and Sweet: A Family's Journey with Cancer" is another inspirational chronicle of a brave fight against cancer. It is also the love story of Tim Colvin and his wife Darcy Thiel in the midst of crisis. Tim was a 48 year old husband and father who was struck down by one of the most deadly of human cancers, gallbladder cancer. Most patients with this cancer present at a stage beyond cure, and most will die four to six months from the time of diagnosis. I am a cancer surgeon who has treated hundreds of patients with this devastating disease and seen so many suffer the fate of the Thiel-Colvin family. This book reminds us of the importance of family and community in such a time of crisis. This book reminds us of the suffering also felt by spouses, children, brothers, and sisters. Cancer is a family matter. Cancer is a family crisis.

The *"Bitter and Sweet"* journey is told through three intersecting narratives. During the 160 days between Tim's cancer diagnosis and his untimely death, Tim and Darcy communicated with their supportive friends and family through a blog on the CaringBridge website. These postings, along with the responses from their friends and family, are interspersed with a reflective narrative written by Darcy a year later. It is as if the present Darcy is in dialog with Tim and their friends in a time passed. Tim's words are like the outlines of his hand left in the cement poured for their pool into which Darcy is now filling with her words. The result is a display of a shared life of love and deeds that transcends time.

Tim and Darcy's story reminds us that life is not just measured in minutes, but also measured in tasks, deeds, and memories. Our lives are both the landmark anniversaries, as well as the routines of everyday life. Life is the family camping trip, the biscuits and gravy on Father's Day, and even chores like fixing the pool or mending the fence. Our sense of mortality comes when we realize we may not finish all that we set out to do. *"Bitter and Sweet"* documents the generosity of many friends and family who volunteered time to help Tim and Darcy in these difficult times. They provided the minutes to complete tasks in the life of a man with finite time.

This book speaks to those of us caring for those afflicted with cancers. If a patient's remaining life is measured in weeks and days, it is imperative that we minimize the inefficiencies that rob the patient and his family of this precious time. The days left should not be spent in the waiting rooms of scanning facilities and treatment areas. The patient should not be spending time speaking to clerks and insurance approval agents but to their loved ones. More time should be spent hugging our children, reading with our spouses, climbing rope courses than with physicians.

This book also speaks to the importance of palliative measures. Many of us will suffer a disease that the doctors cannot cure. It is important at that time to have available all those things that provide relief from suffering: whether it is steroids for appetite, analgesics to alleviate pain, acupuncture for nausea, or massage to allow relief of stress. The traditional medicines, the integrative and alternative techniques, and finally the hospice measures are all important to ease suffering for the patient and his family.

Most importantly, this work affirms that death is not the only certainty. The more comforting certainties are Love, Faith, and the knowledge that "There is much good in this world: much, much, much!!"

Thank you Darcy for sharing your tears, your thoughts, and your experiences so that others may find support and draw comfort during their fight against cancer. I wish for you a long, healthy life and happy memories of your time with Tim.

And Tim, I wish for you great comfort and peace.

INTRODUCTION

When my husband Tim was diagnosed with cancer, one of the things that we did differently was start to read together. We would often take turns reading and as his condition worsened, I did most of the reading. Usually, he would fall asleep at some point and I would bookmark where we left off. We were exposed to some great books. They were instructive and inspiring and helped us tremendously. After his death, I continued to read more. Excellent books on grief abound. I reference some of these books throughout the text.

When I began to give serious thought to writing this book, I thought "Another grief book? Do we really need one?" That was when I realized that one of the dreams for this book, is to be part of another's arsenal. Perhaps our book will be one in a stack of helpful books for someone else — including those who are going through a terminal illness, and those who love them and want to understand how to be involved in a meaningful way.

As we read, we often came across this idea that the tragedy you are dealing with is a gift. Many people evolved to the point where they could honestly say they were grateful for whatever trauma that was brought into their life. Because of the way they had grown or because of whatever benefits they derived due directly to having their infirmity, some even concluded they would not remove their issue if given a chance to.

We never reached that point. We never stopped thinking that cancer is a hideous beast. Tim often said his cancer was "particularly clever" because of the way it hid itself until it was too late. The *"bitter and sweet"* became our mantra. We saw the bitter. But we did truly know and see that there were also gifts in our lives, every step of the way. And we knew that many of those gifts would not have come if it weren't for the cancer. And we were truly grateful for those gifts and felt blessings deeper than anything we had felt before. But don't think for one moment that we wouldn't have forfeited the gifts and blessings if we could be rid of the robbing and cruel disease if we were given a choice. We could have continued down the slow path of evolving ourselves in "normal" life circumstances and been okay with that. Somehow, I don't feel like we missed the boat though. People still experienced us as inspiring on every front, in spite of the fact that we didn't express gratitude for the cancer. There are absolutely silver linings in every cloud, but the cloud is still there.

I can't possibly begin to thank the myriad of people who helped us get through this ongoing event in our lives. God. Angels and spiritual beings. Family and friends (especially my "ya-ya's"). Colleagues, church family, agencies, hospitals, and counselors. It would be impossible to list them all. Mostly though, I must thank Tim, my husband and partner. He was the biggest hero of them all. I'm not sure what you believe about the afterlife, but I have come to understand his presence and dedication to me and our family in a very real and steadfast way *since he has departed from this life*. Thank you my love!

This story is as true as I can make it be. But because the story touches much more than just me, all of the names in the book have been changed with the exception of Tim, myself, and our pets in order to protect others' privacy. While Tim was sick, we were informed about CaringBridge, a website where people can write journal updates to keep loved ones informed. Much of the text of this book comes from those entries and the guestbook entries people responded with. The format is set up so that actual journal entries that were published online are boxed in. Guestbook entries are set apart by shading so you can recognize them when they occur.

My hope, desire, and prayer is that you find this to be an exercise in genuine life — opening yourself to feel the most bitter of human emotions, and then allowing yourself to taste the sweet that comes along side of it. Blessings to you!

Bitter and Sweet:
A Family's Journey with Cancer

Chapter One:
2010, B.C.
(Before Cancer)

March 25, 2010

Have you ever had one of those moments where a million things run through your mind in just a few seconds? I was having one of those moments. I had just taken an exam to be a licensed Mental Health Counselor in New York State. I was waiting for the results, which are printed out immediately after taking the exam. As I stood there, holding my breath, the last 13 months flashed through me.

I have been a couple and family counselor in private practice for almost 13 years. When my son Frankie had entered kindergarten, I thought it was time to work more daytime hours and applied for a position near my home. During that interview process, I was informed that New York State had changed all its' regulations for practicing as a therapist. After recovering from the panic, I suddenly found myself back in graduate school trying to get the requirements fulfilled. School was tough enough the first time, but going back as a wife, mom, home owner and business owner was overwhelming to say the least. Got the classes under my belt, but now I had to pass this exam!

I'm definitely not a great test taker. Just don't like the pressure. I took practice tests and attended a workshop that were very helpful. Our lives had been turned upside down. So as I stood there waiting, I could only hope that I would pass and life could finally return to "normal." The proctor handed me the results without a smile on her face. "Not good, huh?" I said. "Oh, I never look at the results," she responded. A nervous peek. I PASSED! I couldn't call my husband Tim fast enough to let him know the stress was over. Boy, do I like the technology age — no six weeks or months waiting period to discover my fate.

I will gladly take on the next phase of my life — that of building up my businesses again. This detour was exhausting but I am back on track!

1

By the way, Tim and I have been married nine years. We have three children from his first marriage - Emily, who is 29 years old. She is married to Spencer and lives in Georgia with our three year old grandson, Parker. And she is expecting our granddaughter ☺. Colin is 26 and lives with us. Matthew is 23 and lives nearby. And together we share our son Frankie, who is seven years old, going on 22. Life has definitely been full!

April, 2010

I am a person who often has some sort of infirmity going on. Tim is proud of the fact that he is rarely ill. He can eat and eat and eat (even the wrong kinds of foods) and not gain any weight. Everyone told him it would eventually catch up with him. It did a bit around his mid 40's. He has developed a little bit of a basketball around his middle, but overall still looks good. I have had a daily pill box for years. Tim has always been medicine free.

About mid-April, he came to me and said he was having a more consistent "weird sensation" in his stomach. He said it wasn't painful, just odd. But he had noticed that it was hanging around more and more. He decided to make an appointment with our doctor. We love her to death! It was unusual for him to see her so I knew the "feeling" had gotten more annoying.

April 22, 2010

Tim went to see Dr. Grace to talk about his sensations. Grace is a very thorough doctor. She calls herself a "vampire" because she runs so many blood tests if something seems unusual. She isn't over the top, but definitely gives us a feeling of confidence with her attention to the details we talk about.

The clinic notes say "Here for abdominal pain," although Tim preferred the term sensation to pain. It says the pain worsens with deep breaths and that Tim has been worried about his condition. He weighed in at 157 pounds. "Appears healthy and well developed. No signs of acute distress present." All good news.

Treatment plan? Several blood tests are ordered (of course, what else from a vampire?) in spite of the fact that Tim can almost be labeled "needle phobic." He detests them so much, that he avoided a blood test for over a year, even though it could have saved us hundreds of dollars on our insurance! Urinalysis. Standard, I assume. She also ordered an abdominal ultrasound and two chest x-rays. I think her guess is gallstones. If that's the case, they will probably want to remove his gallbladder. It's not a necessary organ anyway, so no big deal. Oh, and "Observe and call if any worsening." Luckily, our doc is quite resourceful. She got Tim in that same day for his ultra-sound.

April 28, 2010

Dr. Grace informed us that Tim indeed appeared to have gallstones and would need to have his gallbladder out. The ultrasound reads something along the lines that the problem may be related to "sludge and stones." That's quite a visual. She referred us to Dr. Wright, one of the best in the area. We chose Grace carefully for her dedication and brilliance. Her referrals are always nothing less.

Tim had his first consult with Dr. Wright today. I decided to attend appointments with him from now on. I have a need to be informed and I think Tim likes having me there. Dr. Wright explained the laparoscopic process. It's all so simple now. Not even any big incisions. He just goes in through Tim's belly button and sucks out the gallbladder. He even made it sound kind of funny. It's a standard operation; doesn't even require an overnight stay in the hospital. Recovery period is only a few days before he should be able to return to work. Tim is an incredibly hard worker and hates to miss it so he's glad about that news.

Dr. Wright had read the ultrasound reports also, and there was a sentence that said there was an "Impression that contained the possibility of a gallbladder mass or tumor... blah, blah... neoplastic process that should be considered." Obviously, that's not a direct quote, but it truly does sound like Greek sometimes. It wasn't terribly concerning, but being a great doctor, he is also thorough. He asks Tim to schedule an MRCP. We've never heard of that before so he explains it's like a super-detailed MRI. Okay, we understand that. It needs to be done at Mercy Hospital. Probably only a half day off work, also a relief. After Doc gets the results, he will schedule the surgery.

April 29, 2010

Tim went for his MRCP test and I accompanied him. We won't get the results until our next appointment.

3

April 30, 2010

Today we went to a Buffalo Bison's baseball game. Frankie was in Cub Scouts and had to walk in a parade there in uniform. It was sort of a good time — it's always good to be with family. But Tim complained several times throughout the game. "I can't wait to have this gallbladder taken care of" became the mantra. The discomfort was clearly steadily increasing.

Matthew and Tim

Otherwise, it was an uneventful night until my father got hit in the face with a flying t-shirt from one of those shooter guns. Nailed him right in the glasses. After a ridiculous chat with the EMTs there, I took him to the emergency room. He ended up being fine, but I knew the paramedics at the stadium did not do anything close to what they were supposed to do. It makes for a good story anyway. I had to chuckle when I filled out the papers in the ER. Under what happened, writing "hit in the head with a t-shirt" seemed pretty funny.

May 3, 2010

Back to the surgeon. It's a relatively quick appointment. The MRCP results show nothing of concern. Whatever the reader saw in the first sonogram is not seen as a concern in this more sophisticated picture. The "impression" could be explained as gallstones. The ducts were not constricted. There is moderate fat in the liver, which often happens with age. What does that all mean? Bottom line —"There is no contra-indication for surgery." We're glad it's a go, but also thankful for his thoroughness. Better safe than sorry, right?

May 5, 2010

Back to see Grace, our family doctor. This time the agenda is listed as "pre-op for laparoscopic cholecystectomy." Geez, why are medical terms so long and impossible to pronounce? Tim weighs in at 156, just one pound less than last appointment. Check. There is a super-long list of questions, all with negative answers. Check. (I guess the medical world is one of the few places where "negative" is actually positive news.) "Medically cleared for surgery. Labs and EKG are

4

within normal limits." Check. This is the first time we see a diagnosis on paper, compliments of Dr. Wright, Tim's surgeon.

574.10 Calculus Gallbladder with Other Cholecystitis without Obstruction.

We don't know what most of that means. But it doesn't seem important to know either. Simple gallbladder surgery. Since telling people about this, at least a dozen people have said "Oh yeah, I had that done, it's a cinch."

Chapter Two:
A Lot Can Happen in 24 Hours

Friday, May 7, 2010

Morning
Today is the day Tim gets his gallbladder out. Then he has his short recovery period and can go back to eating normally. We scheduled surgery on a Friday so he will most likely be able to return to work on Monday. Today is also the day of Frankie's Mother's Day program at school. Surgery is scheduled for the morning so hopefully by the afternoon my Dad can just bring Tim home from the hospital while I am at the school.

You know how things go at the hospital. Delay after delay, little communication. One surgeon, scheduled for many operations, all of which can develop a life of their own.

Afternoon
I end up leaving the hospital and heading to Frankie's first grade classroom before Tim even goes in for his procedure. I'm a little bit nervous, because surgery is still surgery. I see Frankie's friend's mom on the way in. We chat and I tell her I've come from the hospital and will have to return after the presentation. She informs me that she has had the same operation. "No biggie, not even scars. He'll have no problem," she says. I let her know we've heard that a dozen times and we are relieved. Then Frankie and his classmates brighten the day with a poem and song about what great moms we are. I usually stay and chat, but leave quickly to get back to the hospital.

I arrive to find that I haven't missed his surgery at all. He still hasn't gone in yet. Now Dad is relieved of watching-Tim-duty and is reassigned to go-home-and-get-Frankie-off-the bus-duty. Thank God he is around. My family has always been pretty amazing when it comes to helping each other out.

Poor Tim is just so sick of the whole thing by this point. Sitting all day in the hospital, waiting after a few weeks of stomach annoyance and not being able to do his favorite thing (eat!). Finally, about 6:00 PM, they took Tim in.

I was sitting in the operation waiting room by myself. I don't remember what I was doing. I think I was people watching and mindlessly watching TV. I rarely watch TV, so once in a while it's a nice distraction. I don't remember what time it was when Dr. Wright appeared in the waiting room. I know I was surprised that he was done so early, but not alarmed. He motioned for me to come over to him.

He took me into a room and shut the door. I had a slight feeling of panic at the closed door, but quickly dismissed it knowing how important adherence to the HIPPA laws is these days. Generally speaking, I can be very calm, even in a crisis. I keep my head on, pay attention, and ask the right questions. Dr. Wright explained that he was unable to remove Tim's gallbladder. He said they usually go in and suck it out through the belly button, which was the type of incision he made. However, when he got in, he said the gallbladder was hard as a rock. He said it was like trying to take a pair of tweezers and grab a piece of the wall with it. You just can't do it. The "right upper quadrant" was moving together. When he pushed on the gallbladder, everything moved with it because it was stuck together. This indicated possible neoplasticity.

Okay, then, now what? One option would be to pull out and open him up, just like they used to do in the old days. They could get it out, but recovery would be longer as it's a more invasive surgery. However, he didn't recommend that.

He then showed me several color photographs of pictures he had taken of Tim's insides. (Wow, you've got to love technology, even though it wasn't a very appealing picture.) He showed me the color and marks that looked like the canker sores you can get in your mouth, etc. He wasn't sure what it was and wanted to get a biopsy. It was these marks on the surrounding areas that concerned him most because that meant things could have spread already. It was Friday though, and they couldn't run labs on the weekends. I asked him the key question. "You are an experienced surgeon and I realize you cannot say anything for sure, but what is your best guess?" "Cancer" was his response. Now I start to shake. It turns out "neoplastic process" is a nice term for cancer. Technically, it's "an abnormal new growth of tissue." (A pregnancy actually fits this description too, but usually the term has negative connotations.)

We continue to talk. He says the medical call is mine to make. He can go in and take out the organ, or take some biopsy samples and pull out until more tests are done. Holy crap! I'm not qualified to make those kinds of decisions! But then I remember that is why we do our homework so well in the beginning. That is why we pick doctors we can trust. I ask him what he would do if it was his wife. There was no hesitation — pull out. Good enough for me. Later, we were told by the cancer experts how lucky we were to have him for our surgeon. Many would not have made that call and it was clearly the best medical decision. Dr. Wright is somewhat apologetic. This is the first of many encounters we will face where tests indicate one thing, but the actuality of what is happening is entirely different. The best a physician can do, is make a decision based on what the evidence points to. If the preliminary tests had shown anything else, he would have not attempted this surgery in the first place. Ah, to be human.

Evening
Now I am by myself again and completely in a daze. Thousands of movie scenes run through my head. I think to myself how it really is like they say in the movies. You sit in this waiting room and the doctor comes and compassionately and kindly forever alters your life. After a few seconds, I kick into action like I usually do.

First call is to my dad. He asks me if I want him to come back to the hospital. I hesitate, but who am I kidding? Yes, I want him to return. Colin (our 26 year old) is home so he can stay with Frankie. I know Dad won't be able to do anything, but I hate being alone. I call Tim's brother Roger next. We don't communicate with them on a daily basis so I don't know if they are home, but they literally live right down the street from the hospital. Yes! They are home and offer to come to the hospital also. I'm grateful and I know Tim will be also. A couple of calls to my church pals and minister to keep me occupied while I'm waiting for the next thing to happen.

Soon the four of us are in a waiting room on the recovery floor. They are going to bring Tim through, but he's not there yet. I have another conversation with Dr. Wright. He is extremely apologetic, but still has more operations to go. He does not think he will be available when Tim gets out of recovery. The implications of this begin to settle in as I am waiting. I am going to have to be the one to give him the news. Oh shit. How am I supposed to do that?

Finally, we see Tim being wheeled in his bed to his room. He gets a glimpse of us and raises his hand with a "big thumbs up" in triumph. He is elated to have this thing over with. My heart dropped as I knew his elation would soon be crushed.

I went in the room by myself initially. He starts chattering about how good he feels before I can say anything. I sat next to him and tried to talk in the calmest, most unalarmed manner that I could. "Baby, they weren't able to take your gallbladder out." He truly thought I was joking. When he realized I wasn't, he was rightfully aggravated, and then the flood of questions started. I started bumbling around but in a truly gracious moment that I was incredibly grateful for, Dr. Wright appeared in the doorway. I was so ridiculously happy to see him. A wife shouldn't have to tell her husband he might have cancer.

Doc came in and explained everything again. Only this time, he had snagged a picture of what a healthy gallbladder looks like so we could compare. I suddenly understand on a much deeper level. To me, it didn't even look like it could be the same organ. Holy Shit Again. The family had come in by now. Overall, Tim appeared to handle it pretty well. It was clear that we wouldn't know anything until pathology reports came back, and it was clear that wouldn't happen over the weekend. We all did a pretty good job of not freaking out too much. Soon Tim was signed out and we were able to go home.

The middle of the night
We lay in bed chatting for awhile, trying to sort out what we had heard. We didn't want to assume the worst, but we didn't want to put our heads in the sand either. How do you find yourself suddenly lying in bed with your spouse discussing such things? He looked at me kind of sheepishly and said something about how weird it might seem given the circumstances, but he wanted to make love. I actually didn't think it was weird at all. Even though the mood was sobering, it seemed like such a life affirming thing for us to do. So we did.

Several hours later, I was awakened. I wasn't sure what it was because it was a sound I didn't quite recognize. It sounded human, but was foreign to me. I realized Tim wasn't in bed so I got up to investigate.

I found Tim pacing in the kitchen, sobbing. It was a kind of crying I hadn't heard from him before. In fact, I don't think I had ever heard anything quite like it from anyone. It was a man, coming to grips with his mortality. It was gut wrenching and unfamiliar. Fearful. We all know intellectually we will someday die. But this was a man having a visceral experience that cannot be described well. My heart broke with his as I held him. What was in store for us?

Chapter Three:
The Truth
(It Doesn't Always Set You Free)

When you are waiting, days can seem to take lifetimes. I made several phone calls directly to the pathology lab to try and get results, but mostly we had to wait. There was some mix up and the labs went to California or something goofy like that. We found ourselves facing one of the greatest challenges life throws at us. How do you balance all the information? On the one hand, you don't want to be negative or pessimistic. And you certainly don't want to create any self-fulfilling prophecies. On the other hand, you can't pretend reality isn't reality. Fighting is an admirable stance. Acceptance is also equally admirable. How do you ever manage both?

It brought back memories of when we lost a baby in 2001 before we had Frankie. I had gone for my checkup to hear the heartbeat for the first time. There wasn't one, but my doctor told me not to panic (yeah, right) and sent me for a sonogram. The sonogram showed that the fetus was not developing. He suspected I would miscarry but asked if I wanted to wait another week to see what happened. Of course I did. If there was any chance they were wrong, I wanted to wait. This was on a Tuesday. Funny how you remember weird details like that.

Being a counselor, I was well trained to know that men and women process grief very differently. I was about to understand that on a much more personal level. After the news at the hospital, I immediately began to grieve. Whether I wanted to or not, I started to process the possibility that we could lose the baby. I'm not sure if I had an intuitive instinct that the miscarriage was coming or not, but I started to grieve. Tim, on the other hand, refused to believe in the possibility until it happened. To some extent, I admired his positive energy. But the next couple of days became conflict ridden as our different ways of dealing with it were at odds with each other. Tim truly believed that if I was sad and upset, believing that the baby wasn't growing, that any chances the baby had would be lost. So my grief caused him great anxiety and anger. I couldn't blame him, but I couldn't blame me either. It was just impossible information to process.

On that Friday we went out of town together alone. We sat on a rock at the beach and talked about our hopes and dreams for the baby and the future. In our own way, we came to a meeting of the minds and had some precious time together. Saturday morning I miscarried. We made it through but it was a very instructive experience for us. Little did we know we were also being prepared for future difficult medical information.

May 13, 2010

Poorly differentiated adenocarcinoma. There. We had the official lab results. Dr. Wright called me to let me know. Another fancy word for cancer. Poorly differentiated is the part that extra stinks. It means it's a bad case of it. I thanked him for calling and then sat at my desk. Okay, this is the second time now I have been faced with having to tell my husband that he has cancer. How do I word it? How do I bring it up? As I sat with the pit in my stomach, it hit me that I shouldn't have to do that. That's doc's job. As much as I'm sure he doesn't like that part of his job either, it's still his job. Tim will have a boat-load of questions anyway so it's better if it comes from him. I call his office back and ask them if Dr. Wright can call Tim directly. I gave them his cell number and of course they had no problem doing it. I hung up and was relieved, although I didn't relish waiting by the phone for the call that I knew would come from Tim.

Life often throws us those moments where we say, "Are you kidding me?" or "Really?" or "This is like a bad movie!" We were about to have one of those moments. Tim got the call. He happened to be driving home from work. Hindsight is 20/20, but looking back he wishes he would have just pulled over when he got the call. He got the test results and while they are talking... Get this... Tim gets hit by a truck. No lie. Isn't that ridiculous? It was 100 percent the other driver's fault, but what are the chances?

Throughout our years together, we would often banter about driving. I thought Tim drove too fast, too close, blah, blah. He would then remind me that he had NEVER had a car accident in his entire life. That would immediately shut me up. I had several fender benders under my belt and I couldn't argue with his logic. Forty-eight years without an accident. Until today. What a bitch. Tim described it like this: "So, I'm on the phone being told I have cancer when a truck hits me. It's like getting punched in the face and kicked in the balls at the same time. That's special." Couldn't disagree with him there.

Keeping up with family and friends who want to know what is going on is already getting difficult. I talked with one of Tim's relatives who would like to be updated as often as possible. The problem is, he ends up getting upset at the information and the call becomes stressful. In this case, he was furious with the surgeon. In his opinion, it was the surgeon's fault that Tim was in a car accident. I tried to explain that Tim and I work hard not to "shoot the messenger." An accident is an accident. It's unfortunate, but there really is no value in getting angry about it. Besides, underneath that, we are quite sure our anger is really at the disease but you get more satisfaction yelling at a human I guess. It's ok, but it does make it hard to call people that you know are going to end up yelling. Even if they aren't yelling at you per se, it is still so energy draining.

Later that night, Tim hopped on the computer to see what he could find out about "poorly differentiated adenocarcinoma" as it related to gallbladder cancer. The internet is a double edged sword. It's incredibly informative, but sometimes you need to be careful what you ask for. You have to be prepared for the answer. I distinctly remember one page talking about the statistics around prognosis. It said people generally have four to six months left after being diagnosed. That flipped me out and I thought it was ridiculous. I knew Tim had something wrong, but he functioned almost completely normally. I told him kindly that I was done reading internet stuff. It would just cause me needless worry. He agreed, but said he wasn't too concerned because he was fairly certain that he must be in stage I. He felt too healthy and besides, he just knew it in his gut. If this diagnosis was accurate, he couldn't be more than stage I.

Unfortunately, in my gut, I was worried he was at stage IV. I put in another call to Dr. Wright. I assured him I realized that he could not offer an accurate diagnosis, but I also knew he was experienced and could give me his best guess. He obliged and told me he thought Tim was at stage IV. I hoped he was wrong. But there was no reason to share the conversation with Tim. Tim was very hopeful and there was a chance he was right. And if he's wrong, I'd rather have him be in good spirits for as long as possible anyway.

At any rate, with the official cancer diagnosis, we were being referred to Roswell. They are the best cancer hospital in our area and the appropriate place for us to be.

So as we try to figure out the balance between optimism and reality, we are aware that cancer treatment grows in leaps and bounds every minute. Lots of people live long lives, go into remission, and even get cured. No reason to jump to any conclusions. On the other hand, we are primarily influenced by the experiences we have in our lives. Our personal connections with cancer are as follows. Tim's dad died of pancreatic cancer at age 53. Shortly after that, his mother died of stomach cancer at age 59. Obviously, both were very young. It had a tremendous impact on Tim and his three brothers. When his older brother turned 60, it was such a celebration because he seemed to have broken the pattern. My mother was diagnosed with cancer in 2007 and died three weeks later. Three weeks later. Talk about traumatic. So while Tim and I tried to put up a brave and not-overly-reacting front, inside we were terrified.

May 17, 2010

Dr. Wright has received the final pathology reports and has forwarded them to Roswell Hospital. He told Tim to be sure and let him know if there are any other records or information he needs and he will act as quickly as possible for him. Good guy.

Chapter Four:
Now What?

We are off for our first appointment with Dr. Marco. He has a reputation for being one of the best surgeons at Roswell Hospital. Turns out this surgeon plays tennis with our neighbor. My other neighbor works at the hospital. Both assure us we have the best surgeon possible. We anticipated he would schedule a day for surgery to remove Tim's gallbladder as soon as possible.

I had a vision of how the day would go. Tim has been so brave and optimistic. I figured that he might get bad news today and I knew I would have to be strong. I thought perhaps that he would break down. He's been holding up so well, an emotional collapse might be inevitable. And I will be there for him, ready to be his strength.

The clinic notes said so much. "He really has no complaints. No nausea, vomiting, diarrhea, constipation, chest pain, shortness of breath, abdominal pain, difficulty eating or drinking, jaundice. He has some vague discomfort, is healing from laparoscopic surgery." Vague discomfort. I think that is the phrase Tim has been searching for. So it really shouldn't be that bad.

Tim immediately slips into Mr. Engineer mode. Dr. Marco tells us that Tim is in stage IV. Turns out, gallbladder cancer is pretty tricky. It is very rare and one of its hallmarks is that there are virtually no symptoms until you are in late stages. It doesn't really give you a shot. So we ask him how soon he will be able to do surgery and we are not prepared for his answer. He can't do surgery. It would not be in Tim's best interest. This is when we are told how lucky we are that Dr. Wright didn't attempt to do so either. It makes no logical sense to us. If it's infested with cancer, then why wouldn't you want to get it out of your body as quickly as possible? It bothered Tim tremendously to know this infected organ was living inside of him. We aren't sure we fully comprehend the answers, but we are convinced never the less. Tim and the doctor look at the computer screen and discuss the pictures of Tim's insides. They are intently staring and talking in somewhat technical terms, very dispassionately. I'm sitting in a chair across from them. In a surreal sort of way, the information is trying to sink into my brain. No surgery.

As I am watching my husband, I am surprised and relieved at how well he is handling this information. I was not expecting it to be like this. He is in his brain mode and being quite academic about the whole thing. The big question is always prognosis. Doc says calmly five to seven months left. I am trying to take notes on what I am hearing. Then I realize that the room is growing narrow. What is this? I suddenly realize I may not be doing so well. I get the guys' attention and say calmly "I think I'm going to pass out."

The pace of the room shifts. The doctor sprints over to me and starts taking my pulse. He yells for the nurse, who just about runs in the room. My vision is darkening and I'm dizzy. They get a wet cloth and dab my head. Two nurses walk me to the bathroom. I start to cry. I don't really feel like I'm crying, but I can tell my cheeks are wet so I know I must be. I find my voice. "It's not supposed to be this way. I'm not a fainter, I'm a crier. I am supposed to be his rock. This is all reversed." Only I'm aware that it's more like babbling and I'm only half coherent. The staff was wonderful. They kept telling me Tim was fine, that we had a terrible shock thrown at us and my reaction was perfectly normal. It wasn't normal for me. I didn't realize that finding a new "normal" was going to be part of my daily routine.

So now what? If it's not operable, where do we go from here? We were then taken to our next stop which was the Upper GI Clinic. There he weighs in at 151 lbs., eight pounds lower than the date of surgery. We meet Dr. Hahn, who is going to be Tim's primary doctor from this point on. The treatment at this point is chemotherapy. There is one approved line of intervention which runs on a three week cycle, Capecitabine and Xeloda. They would like to enlist Tim in a clinical trial which includes Gemcitabine and Avastin also. She tried to review all the possible side effects and how the protocol would work.

First step would be to do a CT scan to get a baseline before treatment starts. The chemo will not start until four weeks after his surgery as his body needs to heal from the original surgery before handling what was coming. June 8th was our rally cry, the first day he would be eligible to start chemo. Again, the big question was prognosis. If Tim responds to this first line of treatment, the average survival rate is 12-

14 months. What are the chances he will respond? About 70 percent. She did mention to us that she had a patient with the same disease that already lived past two years. That caught our attention. The good thing about this chemo is that it is relatively well tolerated. There isn't usually horrible sickness with it.

We spoke with another doctor. Her notes read that Tim and I were "anxious but realistic about his cancer." I guess that's the balancing game I've already been talking about. She assured us that there was nothing we could have done that would have prompted an earlier diagnosis. There just weren't any symptoms. And thankfully, Tim had already quit smoking a couple of years before. We told them we were planning to go to Atlanta soon for a week and weren't sure if we should go. They said absolutely we should go. In fact, they quite encouraged us to go before treatment started. From there we spoke to a dietician who was supposed to help us with what kinds of foods Tim could eat. (Not so helpful, but she was nice anyway.)

We literally spent the entire day there. It's a well-run hospital from what we can tell. One-stop service, evidenced by the number of appointments we were able to have in one day. We came home exhausted, emotionally spent, and carrying a huge pile of medication, disease, nutrition, and cancer information. Overwhelmed doesn't come close to capturing what we feel.

Sunday, May 23, 2010

One of my best friends in the whole world lives in Chicago. I lived there 11 years before I moved back to the Buffalo area. Anyway, my music hero is Carole King. Ann's is James Taylor. When Ann's husband found out they were doing a combined concert in Chicago, he thought that we just had to be there. He wanted to surprise her and called to see if I was in. Of course I was and promptly booked a plane ticket for a quick weekend. He would have pulled off the surprise if the bill didn't come in the mail. When she found out he spent over $700 for the tickets, she almost killed him! So did I! We love the artists, but are both much too practical to have ever paid that much for one night's entertainment, no matter how good it was.

So here I am a couple of months later, knowing how much was invested in this weekend, but now finding that suddenly life is very different for us. I didn't know if I should go or not. After discussing it at length with Tim and several others, we decided I should go. I was in for a long haul of battling this hideous disease with him and there probably wouldn't be an opportunity like this for a long time. Off I went.

The concert was indeed fabulous. Ann and I were like school girls listening to the music. But more importantly, it was talking in the hotel room that night, trying to come to grips with what lay ahead that I needed desperately. I could admit my fears and inadequacies there when I didn't need to be strong for my husband. And I was able to be with my best friend — the kind you don't need to explain anything to. It was much needed.

Monday, May 24, 2010

I got up to catch my plane back home to Buffalo. I was an odd mixture of feelings. On the one hand, I felt terribly anxious to get back home. I had a deep sense that I am needed there and couldn't get there fast enough. I think lots of moms feel like that. It's just part of our make-up. So it was normal, just more intense than usual. I sat on the floor of the airport, waiting for boarding calls. I wasn't thinking about anything in particular, but as I sat there, the tears began to come down my cheeks. I'm an experienced crier from birth on, but this was a bit different. It was like I wasn't aware of it, but the tears just fell quietly. Couldn't really stop them either. There was a very pretty lady sitting nearby. I knew she was glancing over at me. I didn't want to make a scene, but I couldn't control the tears. I didn't make any noise so unless you were looking at me, you wouldn't have known I was going through my own personal breakdown.

I think I willed her over to me. She looked so kind. And while I felt nothing and everything at the same time, I had a sense that a kind word would do me a world of good. She did walk over and ask if I was okay. I told her an abridged version of Tim's story. Turns out she was a cancer survivor. She just patted my arm, and I was thrilled to know that someone had survived the hideous disease. Pretty, kind lady in the airport, alias a ministering angel sent from God.

Tim had scheduled his baseline scan for the afternoon. At least this appointment is not tricky, just a scan. When I walked in the kitchen door after my flight, I couldn't believe what I saw. Tim had taken the afternoon off for his test so he was there to greet me with a hug. I looked at him and knew something was terribly wrong. He acted fine, but he looked strange. I had never really seen what jaundice looked like before, but I soon put two and two together in my head and knew

18

that Tim was experiencing that. How could this be? I literally had been gone less than 48 hours! How could things have changed so quickly? Now we are glad to be going back to the hospital. We are learning that life can change with a blink of the eye.

Tuesday, May 25, 2010

Back to Roswell to discuss yesterday's scan and where we go from here. Tim is still working as normal, but has more difficulty getting to sleep and tires more easily. Eating has lost its appeal to some extent so he weighed in at 145, a six pound weight loss just since his last visit seven days ago. The baseline scan showed a lesion in the liver, which may indicate the cancer has metastasized that far out. They gave Tim a script for his anxiety to take as needed. Wonder if I could borrow some of that?

As for the jaundice? Seven days ago his bilirubin was at .9. It is now elevated to 7.1! His bile ducts are being blocked by all the sludge around his gallbladder and will need a stent put in within a couple of days. This will have to be done before we can even consider chemo treatment. Roswell agreed to set it up for us at the hospital across the street. They say it's a rather standard procedure and we shouldn't worry. But then gallbladder surgery was supposed to be simple too. We are already known as the couple who asks a lot of questions. I never go anywhere without a notebook now as the information gets overwhelming!

Thursday, May 27, 2010

Tim and I decided to handle this one on our own. We would drive to the hospital together and come home together. I called one of Tim's family members to just put them on alert in case something went wrong. His response was to kind of freak out. He said our negativity was going to cause bad things to happen, that we were being dramatic and expecting the worst. I was sorry I called. We truly were not trying to be dramatic, just realistic. The real life we lived was that something simple could go terribly wrong. We weren't expecting the worst by any means, but we did need to be prepared if we could be.

┌──────────── **Email update to family and friends** ────────────┐

Tim went to Buffalo General at 1:00 PM today. We were assured this procedure was very simple and routine, but we've already come to understand that just about anything

└──┘

can happen. After some confusion with the surgeon regarding what type of stent should be put in, we realized that Roswell and Buffalo General had not communicated properly about what was to be done. When the surgeon started explaining that stents were made of different materials and the kind they use is dependent on a number of factors, we were lost. After some phone calling and pushing on my part they finally were able to proceed. (Why does it always take being a thorn in some medical staff's side in order to get them to do what should have been done already?) When the surgeon explained the possible complications, we were both pretty nervous. About 4:30 PM the procedure was finished and had been successful without complications. We were soooo relieved.

Buffalo General gave us a script for an anti-nausea medication and one for an antibiotic medication in case he developed a fever. Other than that, there were no follow up instructions at all which again proved to be very frustrating.

Tim was initially very sick with some vomiting. They said this would last an hour or two and then he would be fine. By 11:00 PM, Tim had reached his threshold for pain. He finally let me call the surgeon, but another doctor was on call by then. His pain was not normal and the doctor was worried about a rupture. We had to go to the MAC center at 11:30 PM. They finally gave him pain medicine and he immediately went to sleep. Thank God because the pain was getting unbearable for him. They did a contrast scan and thank God there was not a rupture, but he was inflamed. This was probably due to the stent expanding. He was given an anti-inflammatory script and also another Lortab script. We finally arrived home about 4:15 AM.

As I write this at 8:00 AM, he is resting. He's a stubborn guy so he still hasn't decided if he's going to work today (isn't he crazy?) or if we still plan to leave for our vacation later. Of course, please keep praying for us. I was sitting in the ER all night, just thinking about how this kind of madness is the "new norm" for us. I just don't know how to figure out how to live like this. It's beyond exhausting, frustrating, etc. It's scary for me sometimes to be his advocate. I can be assertive when I need to be, but I don't always know what to ask for. Fortunately, my best friend in Chicago is a nurse so she helps me sort things out about what we should be looking for. I just worry that one time I'll find out too late.

So... The only thing that comes to mind is that song by the Four Seasons "Oh What a Night"... (one of Tim's favorites). Blessings your way.

So much for a simple procedure. Just like the simple operation he had on May 7th. One of the hardest things about being a caretaker and advocate is knowing how and when to let Tim be the judge of things. Of course he is the judge 95 percent of the time. But last night, he was in such agony but was insistent that I not call anyone for hours. When do I override him and risk angering him? I don't feel so wise about this new role I'm in.

Friday, May 28, 2010

Tim and I were planning to take Frankie to Jasper, Georgia to see Tim's daughter and her family. We looked forward to it but in light of the situation, we weren't so sure we should be leaving home. The docs at Roswell not only supported us going, but strongly encouraged us to do so. They said the timing was perfect because it was too soon to start chemo anyway. The best medicine at this point was to do something fun and spend precious time with family. So off we went.

Monday, May 31, 2010

The highlight was a day trip to Stone Mountain. Tim and I are both amateur Civil War fans. Our kids thought we would love it there and they were right. One of the attractions was a ropes course of sorts.

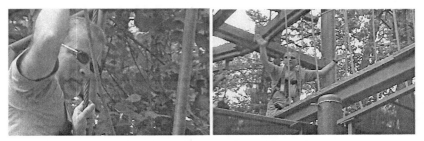

Tim on ropes course at Stone Mountain

21

Tim, Frankie and I all decided to give it a go and went at our own pace. It was so surreal to watch Tim. How could all those doctors be right? He is active and full of life. Could he really be as sick as they say and not have more symptoms? It is so internally confusing.

Tuesday, June 1, 2010

Even though we are on vacation, I realize that I must take a day to make phone calls. Tim is supposed to start chemo in one week. I don't want to lose even one day and I don't want there to be any glitches. I set up shop at Emily's kitchen table with their phone and computer. I quickly realized that I would need to start keeping even more documents in the computer that I can update constantly.

I had no idea what I was getting into. I think I made somewhere in the neighborhood of 35-40 phone calls, trying to follow each lead as far as I could possibly take it. The big issue was Tim's health insurance company. They called me to ask me what his diagnosis is, which I find confusing because I know they have all the same documents and test results I do. Here's the deal. They say that the cancer must have originated somewhere else because they just haven't heard of gallbladder cancer. REALLY? REALLY? I calmly but firmly educate the supposed educated person I am talking to about cancer statistics. Yes, gallbladder cancer is indeed rare. However, MY HUSBAND IS NOT THE FIRST DOCUMENTED CASE IN HISTORY. The torrent of calls and emails that follow is ridiculous. I am in touch with his insurance company, the company he works for, and Roswell. The hospital is trying to provide the insurance company with all the medical research necessary to prove that we aren't making this diagnosis up. Tim's employer is telling me they will resolve this and are mortified this is even happening. I am calm, but forceful. By the end of the day, I realize that it is exactly that - the end of the day. I have spent six hours attempting to be Tim's advocate.

I am exhausted and frustrated and have a ridiculous headache. Meanwhile, Tim is sitting on the living room couch which faces the kitchen I have made into my office. He quietly says to me something like this: "If I am made well, if I get the treatment that I need, it will be solely because of you. I will never doubt your love for me." I would take a thousand more headaches and make a million more phone calls for that man. He made it worth it.

Wednesday, June 02, 2010 7:00 PM
- email update scribed by our friend

Hello Everyone,

Darcy asked me to let all of you know they have received most excellent news from their insurance company today; they have cleared Tim for coverage and the chemo treatment will begin as previously scheduled on Tuesday, June 8th!

Darcy, Tim and Frankie are having an adventurous family road trip home from Atlanta with a stop in Williamsburg. They are still scheduled to arrive home later on Friday evening – God willing and the creek don't rise which they are fully prepared for it to do so given some of the adventures they have experienced along the way – you can ask them to fill you in once they are back home.

Please remember Darcy's request to forward this message to anyone you think appropriate that is not on this listing. Thanks.

For Darcy,
Summer

Thursday, June 3, 2010

We said our teary goodbyes to our kids and headed to Colonial Williamsburg, Virginia. The excitement Summer was talking about? Well, Tim is a mechanical engineer so he has excellent handwriting and map drawing skills. Whenever we take a trip, we have our GPS, but also Mapquest directions printed out, as well as zoomed out maps that are taped together for pages. I always joke with him about it, because we follow the GPS anyway and don't ever use any of the other stuff. So on this trip, Tim conceded and we left New York with nothing but our trusty GPS.

Of course after we left Atlanta, the GPS literally fried itself and was completely dead in the water. We had absolutely no idea what the route was or even when the next maneuver was supposed to be. Boy did I ever eat my words. We ended up calling my Chicago lifesaver and she figured out where we were based on the exit signs, and routed us to the nearest Walmart so we could purchase another GPS.

The other excitement was getting a speeding ticket in North Carolina. One hundred and sixty-four smackers. Tim almost never gets tickets for anything. We had this morbid joke between us about "playing the cancer card." Like, if we told the officer that we had just been given this horrible prognosis and were on our way home from our last trip to see our daughter, and on our way to our last family vacation together, would he really have given us a ticket? Would he be that heartless? But of course we didn't play the card. Just wish we would have.

None of us had been to Colonial Williamsburg before and we had a blast. The weather was sweltering hot but we enjoyed ourselves just the same.

Chapter Five:
Cyber-Angel
(A.K.A. CaringBridge)

Several people encouraged us to look up this website called CaringBridge. It is designed to help people with chronic illnesses (or other such issues) to communicate with others. It seemed like just another time consumer for me with everything else I was juggling. After about the tenth time hearing about it, I decided to look into it, if only to be able to tell people I had. Well, it turned out to be the best resource we had. It was invaluable. To say it was a sanity-saver would not be an exaggeration. I only had to send a link to anyone who wanted it, and they could check on the happenings of our lives whenever they wanted. We named it "The Thiel-Colvin Clan."

• Saturday, June 5, 2010 7:43 AM, EDT

Welcome to our CaringBridge website. We've had so many people tell us about this site so we decided to give it a shot. This way you can check up on things at your own convenience. I will try to update this daily... try being the operative word ☺.

We have finally returned home from our vacation. It was fraught with a million unexpected difficulties (like a very expensive speeding ticket and our GPS dying en route without another map in sight), but we still had a great time. Tim felt well most of the trip so that was a blessing. I will try and talk him into letting me put some pictures up on this thing. He gets a bit nervous

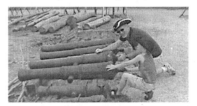

Tim and Frankie inspecting cannons at Colonial Williamsburg

about putting too much information online. We are desperately trying now to get caught up on things. I still have much to organize but we are slowly making progress. Thanks for all your love and support!

Not only were we able to get information out quickly, but there is a guestbook as well. People could sign this at any time. These messages ended up being a tremendous support to us. How many times they brought a smile to our faces, just when we thought we were too exhausted to keep our eyes open.

Another tool that became invaluable was "Care Calendar." I don't even remember how we found out about it, but a dear friend offered to be the "administrator" for it. It was a website that people could log on to. It was a daily calendar where we could list anything at all that we needed. This was when people started providing meals for us, cleaning our house, transporting whomever needed it, and anything else we could imagine. People would sign up, and then get an email reminder when it was their turn. In addition, I got emails every day as to who was providing what service for us. This was yet another most humbling experience for us. All we had to do was ask. People wanted to help in whatever possible way they could.

> • **Saturday, June 5, 2010 6:33 PM**
> **Guestbook entry from my colleague**
> Sending lots of angels and healing energy for you and Tim, and your family. You are all surrounded by love and all things are possible. I will keep all of you in my prayers for comfort and healing.

Being a more traditional "talk therapist," this angel/energy stuff was very new to me, and completely foreign to Tim. I had slowly been exposed to it here and there in my field, as well as from family and friends. I didn't know it yet, but I was about to be catapulted into a journey of exposure about such things.

• **Sunday, June 6, 2010 6:07 AM, EDT**

Hello all, Still slowly attacking our issues/problems one at a time. Of course, it feels like we start one and add another three! Anyhow, some thoughts about needs - our poor Taffy has been quite neglected (our beautiful Border Collie mix we've had for about six months). If anyone likes animals and wants to take her for a walk at the park or creek, or wants to give her a good brushing, let me know! Also, the gals at my church are having a hard time finding people to help out with cleaning. If you are interested let me know by journal entry or email. (Would anyone actually be interested in such a thing?)

Thanks to all of you!

Tim and I made a conscious decision to make our story public. We had come to realize that there were lots of people who wanted to help us, but we had to ask. No one had any clue what we needed, and half the time we didn't either. But we figured we'd just ask as we thought of things and see what happened. The results were astounding.

> **• Sunday, June 6, 2010 7:06 AM**
> **Guestbook entry from my supervisor**
> Darcy, I am particularly here for YOU. I know you may need to talk to someone other than family and friends. Don't hesitate to call...

I hired my supervisor when I started my practice. She has been published and is one of those people who early on, encouraged Tim and me to think about putting our story into book form. It was a crazy idea to us, but also an appealing one.

> **• Sunday, June 6, 2010 7:46 AM**
> **Guestbook entry from my friend**
> I am glad you went on the vacation! Thinking of you and remembering what a remarkable woman you remain and holding Tim and your family deep in my heart.

This woman was my employer turned friend when I lived in Chicago. She was one of those people that invested in you if she found you worthy. So wherever she worked, I went with her. And when she started having kids, I did child care. I had lost touch with her for many years but during my trip to Chicago for the concert, we were reunited over a lovely lunch. Turns out, she has helped many friends go through the journey I was just beginning to experience.

Everyone knows that most people live a circus-like life. Working, child-rearing, house upkeep and zillions of other things have our culture in a whirlwind. We had no choice but to recalibrate our lives with this new information. But why would so, so many others CHOOSE to share in this with us? It is beyond our comprehension.

• **Monday, June 7, 2010 6:24 PM, EDT**

So another day on the roller coaster that is now our "normal" life. Since 8:45 AM this morning I've documented 15 phone calls. (I'm sure there were more that I didn't write down.) Turns out the medical insurance was NOT approved at all. It was a nightmare day. I truly felt like I might have a heart attack, my chest hurt so badly. In the middle of it, I did take a break to meet with my Bible study chums. Good thing because I had a good cry fest with those lovely ladies...

At 5:00 PM I think we got another final "It's all ok and approved" message. I hope they are right this time. At 5:45 PM, I got a call from a Roswell "patient advocate." I explained our situation and also told him I can't possibly have these kinds of six hour days fighting with 5-7 entities (literally!), all giving me contradictory information. I told him I applied for his position last year (obviously I didn't get it) and I needed a strong fighter. I obviously can do the battling myself but it has taken a great toll on me. He promised to impress me, said he is my new lifeline, and he is the only one I have to deal with from now on. He also volunteered to come to Tim's appointment tomorrow morning to ensure it runs "smoothly and perfectly." I cried again, this time for joy and relief...

• Monday, June 7, 2010 6:33 PM, EDT

Oh yeah... I forgot our "needs"... of course you have all already been amazing...

I am out of drink supplies for my office. I usually watch for sales; however, I don't have time for that. So I could use someone who could do a big drink run, usually several cases of water and pop. I write a business check for that... if anyone is interested, please let me know.

• Monday, June 7, 2010 7:21 AM
Guestbook entry from Tim's friend
Coop, I am looking forward to being there this weekend. My deepest sympathy for you and your family. Be strong and always remember that you are loved.

Jim is Tim's best friend from childhood. "Coop" has been Tim's nickname for most of his life. Don't remember the story behind how that got started, but I've grown used to it over the years when Jim comes into town. I remember when Frankie was born and we received a gift in the mail addressed to "Baby Coop."

• Monday, June 7, 2010 8:35 AM
Guestbook entry from Tim's friend
Tim and Darcy, It has been a long time since we have seen you, but we think of you and remember the "old days" fondly. Our family has been keeping you in our nightly prayers and we wish you all the best. Many good thoughts and prayers to you all.

One of the "sweets" in our lives we are growing increasingly aware of, is the rekindled relationships that form as news of Tim's diagnosis spreads. Relationships that had been torn apart are being restored. People that had been forgotten are being remembered.

> **• Monday, June 7, 2010 4:27 PM**
> **Guestbook entry from Tim's colleague**
>
> Hey Tim, Glad we had a chance to chat. You've always attacked every problem head-on, so I doubt you'll approach this differently. You've always struck me as a very independent person (aside from being practically useless without Darcy ☺). As you make your way through this, you'll have to learn that it's alright to depend on others once in awhile. I'm sure also that you're going to have the opportunity to see exactly the kind of impact you've had on those around you. Perhaps like you never would have imagined.
>
> We look forward to seeing you and Darcy again soon. I'll keep in touch so we can make it happen. Or should I say, I'll have my planner meet with your planner. Till next we chat... Take care.

Boy, is he right on. It is an amazing experience to watch Tim see love and support like he never thought possible. It is part of the powerful transformation that is taking shape.

> **• Monday, June 7, 2010 7:48 PM**
> **Guestbook entry from Tim's colleague.**
>
> Tim, Darcy and family, We have been thinking of you and we wish you well tomorrow. I put you on the prayer list at school, so there are lots of "little ones" praying for you. If we still had Campbell and Briere, it might be US raising the Cup on Wednesday!

Campbell and Briere... former Buffalo Sabres hockey players. Our house has a lifetime full of obsessed, passionate hockey fans. It was a foreign world to me when I first met Tim, but I have slowly begun to catch the fever. This writer was not only a colleague, but was one of the season ticket holders with us. In February, we took a mini-vacation to Toronto to the Hockey Hall of Fame. Don't know how we had lived that long without having gone before!

Chris lost his wife at a young age. People do an amazing job of trying
to walk a mile in your shoes. But there is some different connection
with people who have actually walked the path before you. They get it
in ways other people do their best to, but can't always achieve.

She and I work in the music ministry together at church. She also
works at Roswell Hospital so she jumps in to help wherever she can
in that arena.

Chapter Six:
And So It Begins...

Hello all! I'm sorry it has taken me so long to post today; so many of you are anxious to hear how things went yesterday. Suffice it to say we were gone from 8:00 AM to 6:30 PM, at which point I worked until 10:00 PM.

Tim checked in at 144 pounds, only a pound loss from last visit. The good news is Tim started his chemo treatment. He does not seem to have had any ill effects thus far, which is a truly great sign of how things may go with this treatment. We had to get an arsenal of prescriptions and medications to have available in case any side effects do develop.

His chemo runs on a 21 day cycle; he receives two meds thru an IV on day one, then one med thru an IV on day eight; each IV is only 30 minutes, which is relatively short. In addition, he takes pills twice a day for the full 14 days; the third week of the cycle he is completely off. This gives his body a chance to recover before the next round starts.

This cycle is on Tuesdays, but in July it will switch to Thursdays.

The not so great news was that it was a grueling day. Tim had blood drawn four different times; it took them three attempts to get his IV in; and that was the hardest part for him. He is sore in his arms more than anything else.

For me, it was a morning of fighting hard (and crying hard) as the medical staff had decided before we got there that they were not going to treat him until Thursday. We were tracking UPS for medicines and they had to be rushed from our house to Roswell. It was exhausting and trying but we both feel it was worth the fight and turmoil. Bottom line is Tim got treatment and he feels tremendously better on the inside now that something is actually being done. That is the "priceless" part that makes all the emotional agony worthwhile.

Needs? Tim and I have agreed to try and read a couple of books that have been recommended repeatedly to us. They are "The Last Lecture" and "The Triumphant Patient." If anyone has these books to loan to us, we would love it. If not, if anyone wants to research the cheapest place to procure them, that would be helpful as well.

Also, anyone who loves to shop/research online stuff with stores, etc., we need some outdoor things that are time consuming to locate... let us know.

Can't begin to tell you how deeply we love you all!

This is the abridged version of how the day went. I mentioned earlier that I had applied for a patient advocate position once at Roswell. After today's events, I can almost guarantee they would do anything to keep me out of a position like that. What baffled me was the ridiculous fight I had to win in order for Tim to start treatment. You are given this diagnosis and prognosis that there is very little time left. Then they (the medical professionals) act like a couple of days is no big deal. What's the hurry? And I just want to shout "Are you kidding me?"

Our patient advocate gave me the impression by the end of the day that his job was not to advocate for us at all. It was to keep us quiet and cooperative to make the " professionals' " jobs easier. There were obstacles placed before us and I just kept dismantling their arguments, the final blow being my handing them the medicine that arrived at our house via UPS. They had no more excuses and reluctantly set Tim up for his treatment. The "advocate" came at the end of the day to politely tell us that what happened that day was unusual. In politically correct jargon, he basically told me I wouldn't get away with it again. I just smiled angrily to myself. "Just you wait," I thought. "I'm fighting for my husband's life. You haven't seen anything yet."

Wednesday, June 9, 2010

Tim wrote his first journal entry today. I had received an email from one of his family members last night, politely informing me that I was not using the CaringBridge site properly. He was certain that most people who read it were only interested in medical updates. Requests for help should be excluded. It was terribly upsetting to both Tim and me. I decided to leave it to Tim to respond as it was his family. After sleeping on it, he wrote this beautiful and eloquent entry.

• Wednesday, June 9, 2010 12:40 PM, EDT

Hello everyone,
For those of you who have known me for many years, I am Mr. Workaholic – Independent – Do everything for yourself - Ask nothing of others type of guy. Prideful and stoic, I always wanted to be considered the "go to" guy. The toughest part of my illness is that I am now forced to become the opposite of all of those things. For me this has been the saddest part of being afflicted with cancer. For me, it has been sadder than the cancer itself and its potential to take me. It is with this in mind that I have decided to pen my first journal entry.

I thought I'd write about how useful this website has been in relating information to all interested parties, both my medical progress etc., as well as relating the needs of myself and my family, whose lives and structure have been turned upside-down as a result of my sudden and tragic medical condition. I wanted to stress to everyone that we consider CaringBridge to be a multifunctional and comprehensive tool. Although it is quite the nice medium with which to report on the progress of my condition (or lack of progress), I'd like to emphasize that my life is not the only one that has changed. Because I have little or no productivity at home as a "Doer of Tasks," the burden of day-to-day life has increased significantly for my wife and two sons. Not only have they been required to pick up the (my) slack due to my inabilities, but they spend a large percentage of their time tending to my personal needs and wants. For instance, on my inaugural day of chemotherapy we left home at 8:00 AM and didn't return home until 6:30 PM. Darcy then had clients to see from 7:00 PM to 10:00 PM. These are clients that may have already been rescheduled several times and as exhausted as my wife was from seeing to my needs all day, she went out and worked to meet the needs of her clients. Basically, this is all intended to illustrate that because I have become the top priority, that little else is being accomplished.

I hope this justifies why we are also utilizing this website to express our needs as a Family and that it is not misconstrued as an inappropriate means of soliciting any help in meeting those needs. We have received numerous individual emails offering help of any kind and in any way, shape or form.

Because it has become so very difficult to respond to 50-70 emails per day regarding such offers to meet our needs, we have felt that the same method used to apprise everyone of my medical progress (CaringBridge) could also serve as the same vehicle with which we could express our needs.

Here is an excerpt of an email we received from CaringBridge itself, urging us to utilize the journal to go beyond basic health updates:

"Your CaringBridge website has received 269 visits from supportive family and friends! Here are a few tips to help you get the most out of your CaringBridge experience. Update your journal whenever you have news to share. It's ok to go beyond basic health updates."

In order to create more clarity regarding the manner in which our family is taking full advantage of this vital internet resource, we will be issuing future journal updates with an A/B format as follows: A) Tim's Med Update and B) Family Needs. I hope you all find this recital to eloquently explain the need for our comprehensive use of this medium. I want to especially express our gratitude to those of you who have already volunteered to help us — most of whom work full-time jobs, and have families of their own to take care of. I can't thank you enough for your caring deeds and sacrifices and your sincere and heartfelt thoughtfulness.

My final note is to assure everyone that I fully intend to fight for my life, scratching and clawing and kicking. I simply refuse to believe it can take me. My motives are selfish — If I go, you lose one person, but from my perspective, I lose everyone and that is unacceptable to me. I promise all of you, that all of my energies will be channeled towards beating this thing and perhaps breaking mortality records or being the one guy who stumps all of the medical professionals because I won't go away... and that during this journey, I am exceedingly grateful for the new connections I have made and for all the renewed connections as well. I love you all!

Tim Colvin

And indeed, the support was astounding. People sacrificed for us. They gave up income, time, and precious energy to be with us. Tim's attitude was inspiring and I think people wanted to be part of it.

• **Wednesday, June 9, 2010 7:38 AM**
Guestbook entry from my childhood neighbor
Young Frankie is growing fast. I shall pray for some very special happy times for you with your family. Love you lots.

• **Wednesday, June 9, 2010 1:39 PM**
Guestbook entry from our church family
Well MOVE OVER Lance Armstrong because Tim Colvin is going to out race you! Way to go Tim! Now THAT is the kind of attitude, coupled with God and prayer, that will serve you well. In the long run, it may provide the miracle required and if not it will most certainly, beyond any shadow of doubt, leave a legacy of a "way to live" that is indeed life changing for your entire family. Prayers for strength, peace and a huge measure of hope.

These words were prophetic. But then, that has always been Summer's spiritual gift - she is a prophetess from way back. Not only is she a formidable friend, she is a tower of strength, month after month after month. Our legacy truly is beginning.

• **Wednesday, June 9, 2010 3:34 PM**
Guestbook entry from my sister
Tim, your message was eloquent and uplifting. Our support and love are with you whenever you need them. If anyone can fight this, you can.

Hey everyone,
Just wanted to let you all know Tim had a little rougher night last night. He had a slight fever, but high enough to call the doc (per their instructions). They didn't want him to do anything unless the fever persists. He has a little more pain, but the problem is when he takes the pain meds he gets constipated, which then increases the pain... vicious cycle. He also seems to be slowly dropping weight.

He is sleeping mostly upright on the couch recliner now; it has gotten more and more uncomfortable for him to lie in a flat position. We have a person who is letting us look at their adjustable bed as we may pursue getting one to make him more comfortable.

Of course, he is at work today anyway in spite of his night. It wasn't awful, but definitely a shift in how he's been feeling...

Thanks to all of you amazing people helping out so much. We have a copy now of "The Last Lecture." We love you so much!

• Thursday, June 10, 2010 9:45 AM
Guestbook entry from our church family
Hi Tim and Darcy, As your official "housecleaner coordinator," I have lined up another volunteer. That will give you cleaning coverage twice this month. Let me know which day is best and I will contact them to confirm. Others have also offered their help. Loving thoughts to all of you.

• Thursday, June 10, 2010 11:06 AM
Guestbook entry from our church family
Hey Tim and Darcy, Just wanted to let you know I have been thinking about you. Hearing how positive you are made me so happy! I am praying for you. Keep thinking those good thoughts — you know what they say about the power of positive thinking, not to mention prayer.

My least favorite ride at the carnival is the roller coaster, yet ironically it seems that is exactly what I have been on for the past couple of days. But for the most part, the majority of that ride has been high points. Thursday the 10th, I napped after work until 8:30 PM, got up, ate supper, took my chemo dose and went to bed until morning. All that rest must have been just what I needed, because I had a fantastic and productive workday on Friday and I felt very good all day long. Typically I do much better after my morning dose of chemo, than I do with the evening dose. Friday the 11th, featured an uneventful evening. After a minor glitch (pain) at 2:00 AM that had me up to take a pain med, I slept the rest of the night. Saturday morning, I took Frankie to his baseball game where he excelled as usual. Near midday, my friends arrived to visit me from Michigan. They spent the afternoon hanging out. Their cousin also dropped in... as did my brother who was at my aunt's house in the neighborhood getting his haircut. My son Matthew, who has been spending much more time with us lately, also stopped by. At night we walked to a pub for dinner and afterwards said our teary goodbyes. Only one more pain inconvenience last night involving reaching for my pain and anti-nausea meds, but that's about it.

I am looking forward to having a good Sunday today before diving back into the throes of the upcoming workweek. As you can see, it has been mostly good as my body's learning curve for coping with the chemo treatments seems to be coming to an end, now that I am getting accustomed to it.

My thanks and gratitude to all who have continued to be our angels last week, who have shopped for us, cleaned for us and fed us, and who have done it all so very nonchalantly and as naturally as breathing. You are all my heroes and I am humbled before you all.

I will make subsequent entries as the workweek progresses, with the lofty goal of continued success with my ongoing treatments and good news to pass along as well.

My love to all of you,
Tim

Oh my dear Tim, well said. You are *my* hero.

We are supposed to be putting up a fence around our pool on Saturday, June 19th. Tim can manage the project but can't do the actual labor. Tim's "bucket list" has been small and simple (so far). He wants to spend his potentially last summer by our repaired pool, the last part of which is finishing the fence.

I was able to round up a couple of people, but we had hoped for a few more men to lend their strong arms. So "we're looking for a few good men"… and we will need something to feed those big, strong guys…

Please let us know ASAP if you can help or know someone who can; we really appreciate you!

Tim and I are avid home re-modelers. We have been in our house for nine and a half years. Most of that time we have been redoing something - inside or out of the house. We work hard to avoid debt and have been relatively successful. Our pool had originally been poured in 1958. It is an inground, 20 x 40 foot pool and in good shape. It does need some work though. We did our research and finally had a plan that would be divided up over three years. We are finally ready to start phase one. When Tim was diagnosed, we had several conversations about this. Was this the wrong time to even start such a project?

Tim decided that he truly did have a small bucket list. He didn't have an urge to travel anywhere. What he really wants, is to see the pool completely finished. It is our last "big" project and we have been dreaming about it the whole time we have lived here. It seems financially foolish with all we were facing. And yet, we literally have no debt. We are fast learning that life is fleeting. So we made a bold decision that yes, we will start the pool. In fact, we forgot the three year plan entirely. We financed the entire project. It seemed like such a small, small wish to grant Tim — that he be able to lay on his new pool patio and watch his son swim for the summer. Once we decided, we moved ahead. We refused to worry about the money or what other people thought.

It is never about "keeping up with the Joneses" for us. It is about working together and living in a space we can take great pride in.

When someone would come to see us for the first time, I would watch Tim give the grand tour and feel so warm inside. He was so proud of how hard we had worked. And as corny as it sounds, it is truly about being hospitable to others, about sharing it with other people. We often have house guests and many, many of our loved ones know there is no need to ring a doorbell when they come to the Thiel-Colvin place.

One of my favorite memories is when Tim had his entire engineering department over. Every year they are given tickets to a Buffalo Bill's game. We live close to the stadium so the tradition became coming here for pizza and beer first, then I would drop them off at the game and pick them up so they didn't have to struggle with parking. The first year, Tim took those guys around to show them the lay of the land. We had recently redone the guest room. When he got there, he pointed out all the details he could remember. He pointed to the small table next to the bed and said "So we tried to think of everything possible to make someone comfortable who might stay with us. That is why we included this box of tissues by the bed, along with the remote for the TV." And those guys just nodded and smiled. Tim was a regular Martha Stewart.

Chapter Seven:
Round Two

Tuesday — this started the second week of chemo treatments. Thankfully, none of the hullabaloo (is that how you spell that?) from last week. No weight loss today ☺. However, they had to attempt the IV three times again. They blew out a vein in both arms. Apparently, Tim's veins have lots of "valves" so they suggested a mediport be put in.

This will be scheduled sometime next week. It is a simple outpatient procedure where they put a small disk in his upper chest that stays there. Then they simply poke into it for future IVs. We shared the chemo room today with a lovely woman with breast cancer. She has a port and says it is absolutely the way to go.

So Tim is a bit tired out tonight. And once again sore from all the poking and prodding. (He's a little irritable too but don't tell him I said that!)

Another FYI — I have recently spoken with Frankie's teacher, principal, nurse, and social worker. I guess he is somewhat vocal about his dad's cancer at school. I'm actually relieved to hear that because he hasn't been processing this much with us at home. So I'm glad he is feeling safe at school to do so. Plus I know he's in EXCELLENT hands there. Everyone has been totally sensitive and in tune with us and obviously care a lot about our young Frankie.

We love you — and thank you again for all the love and support that comes in so many, many shapes and forms ☺.

• **Thursday, June 17, 2010 12:18 PM, EDT**

Thursday — chemo seems to be taking its toll; Tim worked Wednesday all day but I could tell from his voice he wasn't feeling well. He came home and spent the evening sleeping/resting again. He seems to have more bouts with pain. They come on without warning and are intense. He takes his pain pill but has to wait until it kicks in.

Today Tim called in sick, I think it is the first time since this all started. He doesn't have a fever but he visibly looks like he has the flu — he is exhausted and very fatigued.

On the bright side, they are actually doing work on our pool. It has seemed like a long wait. Tim is very anxious about this and he says this is #1 on his "bucket list." He dreams of doing this last house project and being able to rest on the patio. He had Frankie and me put our handprints in the drying concrete next to his. Then he tenderly told me, "Any time you need to hold my hand, you can just come here and put your hand right in mine"... Yeah, I'm crying again just writing this.

We love you all and feel your prayers and love and support and encouragement. What would we do without you?

42

Actually, the rather large crew of men working (both the concrete and pool crews) had all paused to watch us do our handprints. Several of them walked away sniffling when they heard Tim's motives behind our doing so. Quite a moving day.

• Thursday, June 17, 2010 2:39 PM
Guestbook entry from Tim's colleague in Texas
Tim and Darcy, I want you to know that we at the plant are praying for you. We have thought of you often since you left our company and have loved the occasional updates. Our thoughts and prayers are with you.

• Thursday, June 17, 2010 10:27 PM
Guestbook entry from Tim's colleague in Texas
Tim, It's me, a true friend from Texas. I just heard the news today. I will most definitely put you in my prayers. I still think of you often. You are the most thought of Yankee friend I ever knew, and your contribution to the company will never be forgotten by me. I have always had the utmost respect for you and the job you did for the company. From A True Texas Friend.

At Tim's previous job, he had to go to Texas at times. When we first started dating, I accompanied him on one of those trips. I had never been to Texas before. Tim loves his friends there, and they obviously love him. We decided we need to make another trip there, as soon as he feels able to handle the flight.

• Friday, June 18, 2010 12:53 PM, EDT

Tim went back to work today and seems to be feeling much better... he's such a trooper!

• Monday, June 21, 2010 2:53 PM, EDT
Journal entry by Tim
June 20, 2010 Father's Day Entry
Hello everyone. This may take a few minutes, so get back up, grab your coffee, and then come back to read my journal entry. What a great day I had... three days in a row, Friday,

Saturday and Father's Day. I felt relatively spry and energetic while occasionally fatigued. As much as this particular day is dedicated to trumpeting the virtues of fatherhood, and you'd then picture a Dad, pitching a baseball to an eagerly awaiting son, it has become more about the virtues of the women in my life, past and present. Friday evening, I was handed a Father's Day gift in advance — a plaque about all of the things that cancer cannot do to a man. My former wife surprisingly provided this gift to me. She had it made for me on behalf of my children, who presented me with it.

So now it gets better. On Saturday morning, I was awakened by the voice of my daughter Emily, who lives in Georgia — except she wasn't in Georgia, she was right there standing next to me. It seems Darcy got this last minute idea about how wonderful it would be for me to have all four of my children here with me on Father's Day. In less than 24 hours, she conceived of an idea, made a phone call, got online and just like magic, my daughter was right there in front of me, reaching down to hug me (with my granddaughter inside of her no less). Needless to say, I became temporarily teary eyed at the sight. A half hour later, I found myself in the shower weeping openly and out loud. This Father's Day tribute was most certainly not about me, but rather about just what an amazing woman and wonderful wife I am blessed with. I wept partly because I doubted how worthy I was, to be the recipient of such an incredible gift and to be the husband of such a wonderful wife. Hearing me, she came and consoled me and reassured me that I _was_ absolutely worthy of what had happened, along with all of the other good things that happen to me in an uncertain life.

I was waiting on the couch at 6:00 AM with the camcorder in my hands. I wanted to capture him seeing Emily on video. He was indeed surprised, but didn't have the response I thought he would. It wasn't until a half hour later when I heard what could only be described as lamenting, coming from our bathroom door. It was not that Tim wasn't deeply moved, it was exactly the opposite. It was overwhelming for him. I stripped my clothes faster than a speeding bullet and jumped into the shower with him, finding him sitting on the seat with his head buried in his hands.

"I just can't leave all this love," he said. I just held him and wept with him.

My home became the Father's Day emporium this year, as we hosted a variety of family members who all went out of their way and tweaked their plans to come here, and by doing so, have accommodated (and they do this all the time) my illness and any accompanying discomfort I may have been subjected to in traveling myself. My sister-in-law mentioned in an email the day before that it would be a grand day, and a grand day it was indeed. It started with biscuits and gravy for breakfast. At 11:00 AM, family started to arrive. For part of the day, it was the usual type of get together — girls in the kitchen, preparing food, drinking wine and chatting, and the guys in the living room with golf, Nascar and Space Balls on the tube. We ate our meal and spent a lot of the afternoon taking lots of photos. I got a really cool hockey stick coat rack that I plan on keeping in the sports bar. After everyone left, we took my daughter to the airport for her flight home, stopping along the way for some ice cream at the Red Caboose on Union Road. All in all, it was as grand a day as a Father could have. Very memorable! Having all of my children here was certainly one of the highlights, in a day filled with many highlights.

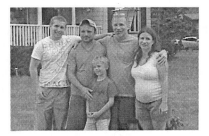

Tim and his four kids

In a subsequent journal entry, if there are any needs we may have, those will be so noted. In closing, I wanted to express our deep gratitude to all of the hardworking volunteers, who sacrificed an otherwise beautiful weather day on Saturday, to come over in droves to get our backyard fence installed. There were men who worked on the fence — a very, very physical task to perform under the hot sun. There were supporting crew — men and women who brought food over, helped with meals and helped by going out and checking on the needs of the laborers. They also cleaned up, made themselves available for errands and helped in many other uncountable ways. My sons and daughter chipped in by running Frankie to his ballgame and birthday party as well as tending to a list of yard work needs — all heroes who "stepped up" and gave of their time and resources to help us. Oh, I almost forgot. Who do you think orchestrated this massive turning out of people power? Again, that would be my wife Darcy, who just when I think doesn't have any more in the tank, seems to have this uncanny persistence of heart and mind, to make the impossible into the possible. I love you, honey! Happy Father's day to all of the partners and spouses and children who make it their quest to keep the Fathers happy — and not just on Father's Day, but every day of the year.

All my love and gratitude,
Tim

It was blazing hot on Saturday, in the 90's I think. I kept thinking of an Amish barn raising, because that was what this was like. It was a community fence raising. These guys worked a good eight hour day, literally dripping in sweat. I watched it go up panel by panel. Tim would go out every once in a while when he felt up to it, just to be part of it. He had put up a million panels of fencing all around our property prior to this. I'm sure it was a bitter-sweet feeling for him to be there — watching, being grateful and amazed, but sad knowing he just wasn't physically strong enough to be a part of it. This will be a day and weekend we will always remember.

• Monday, June 21, 2010 10:53 AM
Guestbook entry from Tim's former in-laws
Dear Tim, Darcy and family, I admire you for the way you have always dealt with any situation that comes your way.

• Monday, June 21, 2010 2:59 PM
Guestbook entry from Tim's best friend
Coop, It was great talking with you this weekend. So glad you got the fence done. The family pictures look wonderful. You should be very proud of everyone. Darcy, great job keeping Coop's spirits up. I am looking forward to seeing everyone again in July. Coop, stay strong my friend and I'll see you soon.

───────── • **Tuesday, June 22, 2010 9:34 PM, EDT** ─────────

Another eventful day on the Thiel-Colvin roller coaster. We arrived at Roswell at 7:00 AM for Tim's mediport procedure. He was getting blood drawn while I was registering him. While I was walking over I felt a funny thing on my leg. I looked down and hanging out my pant leg was a dryer sheet. I started laughing so hard and showed the woman behind the computer but she didn't seem to think it was so funny. Eventually though, I found out she thought from a distance it was a maxi pad hanging out, which is why she didn't think it was so funny. She said "I thought good Lord — first thing in the morning? I am NOT dealing with this woman." So we all had a VERY hardy laugh after that.

Then on to the hospital unit, a place we hadn't been before. I sat in the waiting room thinking "I really don't like this place, it's very unnerving." I was listening to a repetitive loud speaker message saying "code blue" then eventually a "cancel code blue." Now I don't know if you know what that means, but I assumed it meant someone had flat-lined. So I thought "Well, at least they saved whoever it was"...

Next thing I know, this woman approaches me and says "Don't worry, your husband is ok" so I freaked out of course and she took me back to him and he had FIVE nurses working around him. I truly thought I was having a heart attack again...

So, turns out "code blue" means emergency, not necessarily death call (nice to know). Once again, they could not get an IV in Tim's arms and blew two more veins. Tim's eyes rolled to the back of his head and he almost passed out but they were able to keep him conscious. Next thing you know, his PA comes from the other part of the hospital because she had been paged that Tim had a seizure (which was not true). What a scary circus, and the pain in Tim's face was the most agonizing part to me.

Once all the drama was over, he was taken back into the procedure room. They went straight for the jugular (literally) and put the meds in there. The actual mediport only took 10 minutes to install (into the jugular vein) so in the end it was a successful procedure. When Tim started telling dirty jokes I knew he would be ok. (If you want to know specifics you'll have to call me.)

He's very sore and stiff now. It is seven to ten days of inconvenience, but we can live with that. Today he started his week off from chemo and he is loving that idea.

We spent the afternoon arguing about stupid stuff as we deal with the stress we face every day. We're still exhausted and I still feel overwhelmed. Anger is starting to hit which isn't so fun but we keep plugging away at this thing called life and appreciate, as always, all the love and support you send our way ☺.

Tim is well known for his sense of humor. In reality, he is a pretty conservative guy. But when he jokes, he is the most outrageous and unscrupulous man ever. When my mom was alive, he used to offer to take her to her mammogram appointments and assist as needed. When he was unemployed he talked on occasion about becoming a mammogram technician. He loved to shock my niece by asking her to skinny dip.

When he started to lose weight, we were having difficulty keeping up with finding clothes for him that fit. One afternoon, both of my sisters were here and we decided we needed to go through his wardrobe and figure out what he had to work with. So the four of us were in the bedroom and Tim was trying things on as they were shot at him. Suddenly, it hit him. "Hey, I just realized you are fulfilling a long standing item on my bucket list. I am here, without my pants on, in my bedroom, with both of my sisters-in-law. The only thing is, Darcy is NOT supposed to be in here!" Everybody cracked up. Well, everyone but me. I was deeply offended that I wasn't part of the fantasy ☺.

So when I went back to the hospital room and saw him with all those nurses around him, his dirty joke was this. He told me that the nurse that took him back to shave him, was touching herself while she was doing it. I affectionately told him he is an ass.

• Wednesday, June 23, 2010 6:48 AM
Guestbook entry from my supervisor
Darcy, As the anger comes, think of the dryer sheet! Anger and laughing don't usually mix well!

• Wednesday, June 23, 2010 9:59 AM
Guestbook entry from our church family
You and Tim are both so strong and capable. Dryer sheets, dirty jokes — keep laughing and praying. Love ya.

• Thursday, June 24, 2010 3:32 PM, EDT

So... up, down... I'm getting sea sick... my head is LITERALLY spinning...

Up — good old grandpa took Frankie to get a new bike yesterday; it is great! His knees were hitting the handlebars on his old one...

Down — found myself in a waiting room (all too familiar these days) awaiting test results, and hoping for good news. This time it was the vet's office; our very loved cat Oreo has been losing weight. You'll never guess — yep, cancer. You'll never guess — yep, only has a month left if we're lucky. Had to tell Tim and Frankie the news.

Did I mention anger? It is really mounting now. I'm sooo sick of cancer; can I just have one day when it doesn't hurt my family???

Up — Frankie, Tim and I went to Gilda's club last night and did everything we needed to in order to be signed up. We did it mainly because Frankie wants to attend a day camp there in July. Tim showed some interest in a meditation group and also a cancer support group. There's stuff for me in the fall once Frankie is back in school.

Down — Tim woke up this morning and noticed a very agitated lesion; went to work but had to go for an unplanned appointment to Roswell. He weighed in at 139, another drop in weight but it's not monumental.

Up — everything is ok. Nothing cancer related. Plus they changed his bandage while he was there which means I've been able to avoid that today, makes me nervous to be in charge of that stuff.

Soooooooooo, blah, blah, it is a merry-go-round, but half the time it is not fun at all.

Sorry for the negativity, I promise it is just a phase ☺.

• Thursday, June 24, 2010 3:02 PM
Guestbook entry from Mom B
Tim and Darcy, All of the ups and downs make us realize that all is not fair in this journey that we are on. Let's hope that the ups win! Love and prayers.

One day, Frankie and I decided to go to the zoo with my friend and her two kids. It was an activity we try to do once every summer. So maybe doing something "normal" will make life feel normal, even for just a day. We drove together because it's a small hike and parking is an issue sometimes. The plan worked well for part of the day. Then the phone rang.

Tim was at work, but decided he just wasn't feeling good and needed to go home. He said he felt well enough to drive himself, but I could tell he was struggling. He didn't want me to rush home so I tried to continue on with the day's events. The anxiety crept in pretty quickly. I had to be home. I needed to be home. I looked at the kids and gave them the disappointing news. They were all good sports.

The anxiety mounted quickly. We just couldn't get to the car quick enough. My friend couldn't drive fast enough. My throat was starting to constrict. Several lessons learned. Number one, never ever drive together with someone. I have to understand that life can turn on a dime and I need to be able to leave any situation quickly. If we had driven separately, the kids could have stayed longer at the zoo. Lesson number two, don't ever, ever think your life will be "normal" again. Ever.

• **Thursday, June 24, 2010 6:24 PM**
Guestbook entry from our church family
Tim, Darcy, Colin and Frankie, We are so thankful you have such an incredible support group to help with your needs. Keep your faith and please feel the love that is being sent your way.

• **Saturday, June 26, 2010 9:37 PM**
Guestbook entry from our church family
Great family pictures! Sorry about Oreo. I understand the anger — you just start to feel beat up constantly and you just need a break. Well, celebrate the breaks you get from the stress even if it lasts a few minutes — you all need it. We are so busy at Roswell on some days and we get silly and laugh so hard that we all cry. It feels so good. Must be some endorphin release. Tim, it sounds as though you had a wonderful surprise on Father's Day. Cuddle with Oreo!

• **Thursday, July 1, 2010 4:49 PM, EDT**

So... long time, no update; sometimes no news is good news ☺. Saturday, Tim's former in-laws/family came over and brought some food and drink. His former wife Sheila came along with all three of her sisters; this was spearheaded by Vera, who is Sheila's mom. They all seemed to enjoy being re-connected and Tim was touched by the love and concern they all expressed... Thanks to the Schwartz clan!

When I first met Tim, he had been divorced for five years. He had the house and custody of the three kids. But their divorce had been long and bitter. Being a marriage counselor, I was not surprised by this. I have seen even the most civil of people get entirely out of hand when going through the rigors and pain of a divorce. You could see the toll it had taken on the entire family. Over the next several years, we worked very slowly, but very surely to try and heal those memories. It was no easy climb, but eventually everyone began to interact again. The culmination of that hard work came in 2006 when Emily got married. We had the rehearsal dinner here at our house and the ceremony was at the church Tim and I attended. Emily was able to have both of her parents attend all events with civility and even warmth at times. As I watched them all spend time together in the backyard this weekend, I was grateful that we had put the effort in. Time does heal wounds. Hard work heals wounds. And a terminal illness puts it all in perspective.

Tuesday I had my mole removed. No pool for two weeks. I could have cried. They finally finished the pool and now I can't swim... poor me ☹.

Today is Thursday and Tim's brother Garrett took him to start his next round of chemo (thanks big brother!). The doc said his blood levels are excellent. There was some waiting to be done, but Tim said "This chest port is a beautiful thing." Once they got started all went smoothly. His weight was even up to 142.

There are no immediate side effects, so we will wait to see how this round goes; we just take things one step at a time. Last round it was days two and three that were tougher so keep him in your prayers - I know you always do ☺.

P.S. On a side note, our grandson Parker overturned a yellow jacket nest and got stung eight times! Poor little guy... no allergic reaction though so he's recovering well.

stood up for us to be able to do our jobs and you would not give up until it was right! Therefore I know you are strong enough to stand strong for this trial you face. You are not alone in God's hands and a complete circle of friends from the old days here in Texas, who are praying for you and thinking of you each day. We love you and still think of you as a wonderful friend. With the utmost respect for the fighter I remember.

• Saturday, July 3, 2010 11:55 AM, EDT
Journal entry by Tim

So today is day three of my second chemo cycle. Typically, day three is the bad day of all the days in the cycle, but for whatever reason, I woke up today feeling <u>full of life</u>! Ironic, I know. I got up, ate and went out into the yard with Darcy and took care of a few items on our to-do list, as did she. It is a beautiful, sunny and warm summer day. We also took some photos of the completed pool and fence. It even looks better close up! Thanks again to everyone that helped us to achieve this goal during all phases of the project!

We do have a couple of minor tasks (some painting and edging) remaining, that we are struggling to get to. So anyone that may feel compelled to come and help us out again, please contact Darcy. I'm sure she will tell anyone that calls, that the pool is available to cool off in. Anyone is welcome to stop by for a dip, whenever they want to. I would certainly welcome the companionship.

Hopefully, as this current chemo cycle runs its course, these reports will continue to remain as upbeat in nature, as this one does today. Thanks for your continued prayers and for playing such active roles in our lives.

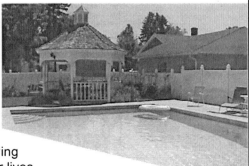

Tim

I don't remember how and when we heard about it, but the chain restaurant Friendly's will do fundraising benefits for causes they deem worthy. You schedule a day and time, and they pretty much do all the rest. You get 10 percent of whatever their sales are during that time period. They provide the flyers and advertisement. There is no set up or clean up. People can eat and order whatever they want. And we are allowed to sell 50/50 tickets. Seems like a very easy thing to pull off. Our friend and "Public Relations Expert" can handle everything from Maine thanks to the internet!

Will everything really get better? And do we even define what that means anymore?

July 4, 2010

The last holiday we celebrated was Father's Day and boy, it would be impossible to beat that. Holidays are already loaded most of the time, but now there is even more added pressure. What if this is the last (fill in the blank) that Tim has when he is feeling well? That was the inspiration behind flying Emily here for Father's Day. Now it is the 4th of July. We decided to spend the day with one of Tim's family members at their cottage. It's a lovely place about a mile from the lake. We usually walk down to the beach to watch the fireworks because there is little or no parking there. Tim and I discussed it at length and decided that in spite of the annoyance, we should not walk the mile there and back. His strength comes and goes and is often unpredictable. We knew his family would not want to drive, so we made our pact before we got there.

The weather was lovely. Things were great until it was time to go to the beach. Tim caved to the pressure to walk rather than drive. I got the impression that my concern was not welcomed by Tim's family, like I was trying to boss Tim around. It was upsetting because they didn't fully understand Tim's physical limitations. Of course, Tim wanted to save face with everyone and not admit that his abilities were compromised. Things were extremely tense between Tim and I. I went to the lakeside so Frankie could swim and just cried while I stood there alone. What if we don't ever get a do-over? What if we have spent our last 4th of July together fighting?

On the way home, some of the family were arguing. By the time the mile walk home was completed, there were tears. We tried to interrupt the fighting to say goodbye but we couldn't break in. We got in the car and Frankie asked what the heck was going on? Tim fumbled an answer about how sometimes people get upset and say things that they wish they hadn't and don't really mean.

We ended up spending an entire counseling session processing this event. Tim and Scott (our therapist) concluded that Tim kind of gets out of sorts sometimes when he's in certain situations. It reminds him of where his own temper can take him if he doesn't work hard at controlling it. We were sad, but are hoping that we get a chance next year to have a more positive and happy 4th of July celebration together. I'm sure Tim's family wants the same. Maybe we can even rival Father's Day!

• Thursday, July 8, 2010 5:51 PM, EDT

Today is day eight of the chemo cycle. Tim's brother Garrett took him to Roswell to get his IV infusion. He weighed in at 139. He is home now and doing ok, no complaints or mishaps this time so hopefully we're starting to get this thing down ☺.

- **Sunday, July 11, 2010 10:51 PM**
Guestbook entry from Tim's family's friend

Dear Tim, I was so sorry to hear about your illness. As you probably know, my husband passed away in February after a valiant three year battle with brain cancer. CaringBridge was a God send to us as we met so many families facing the same struggles that we were... we became friends, family, prayer partners... united by a devastating disease but also by the hope and faith we shared. I know you will find that here too.

Every cancer is different but the enemy is the same. Your journey will be different from ours but please keep me in mind as a resource or just a good listener. I do know what it is like to hear those words "You have cancer." I also know it is possible to beat the odds, live a good and full life with family and friends and to celebrate the blessings you discover along this difficult road. There will be many blessings you never thought possible.

The first weeks and months are very trying and frightening. There is so much information to take in, practical things to take care of, and your family to think about. Let others be your strength. God has sent them to you to help carry your load at this time. Don't be afraid to ask and be specific. God is with you always... on the good days and especially on the bad ones.

Just as quick note about Roswell... we LOVED them... from the doorman to surgeons they were genuine, caring people who came to know us as a family and gave us their best. They touched each of us along the way... treating us with excellent care for my husband but also gentleness, respect and understanding for the kids and I. I will keep in touch through the website but know you or your wife can call me anytime... day or night. Love and prayers.

Our loved ones would tell our story to their friends and family, and our support system just kept growing. There is also a special bond with those who have walked a similar journey. Even though you have just met them, there is a strong connection immediately when you know they have survived what you are only embarking on.

56

Hey all... We just finished reading "The Last Lecture" last night. We admit that we kind of felt disconnected throughout the middle of the book. But the beginning and ending were read with many, many tears and deeply emotional moments. It's a new habit we have... I read to Tim at night before we go to bed. It has provided us with some amazing moments. Our next book will be "90 Minutes in Heaven."

Tim and I were truly transforming our relationship in many, many ways. Reading together was one of those ways. Every once in a while throughout our ten years of marriage I would ask him to read with me. Of course they were topics men aren't usually interested in — like "What to Expect When You're Expecting," or some marriage self-help book and he would not-so-graciously decline. Now we find we really love this time together. Tim can tire easily so eventually I just do most of the actual reading out loud rather than taking turns. This book was the first of many we read.

Hello friends and family!

So today is Tim's first day off chemo; he has one week without it which he always looks forward to; he was a bit more nauseous this time, but overall it seemed to go by more quickly than the first round did.

I got my stitches out yesterday, no cancer, thank God because I think that would have pushed us over the edge. We got our new bed yesterday. It is the first time we've been able to sleep together since this whole thing started. Tim is able to adjust the bed into positions where he is not in pain, yeah for us! Only thing is our king size comforter is too small. If anyone has a king size bedspread or comforter with a bed skirt that is tucked away in a closet somewhere, let us know! Otherwise, we are making do ☺.

As always, thanks for all those meals, support, childcare, etc. We appreciate you all!

This week off of chemo, Tim has felt a bit more ill than he did last time. All in all, we are very excited about the week. Tuesday, we are meeting with a former Roswell patient who has graciously agreed to meet with us. She is now getting treatment in Pittsburgh. She is in her THIRD year of survival with this diagnosis — that is almost unheard of! So we can't wait to pick her brain ☺.

Our very first appointment at Roswell, Tim's doctor told us about this woman. We asked her then if they might ask the patient if we could contact her. Gallbladder cancer is rare so we really wanted to have the connection. That was back in May. Since then, I have called and called and called. Being a counselor, I am aware of the HIPPA and privacy laws. They could not give me her name and address, but they could call her with no problem whatsoever and give her our names and address. The run around I got was crazy. But in my relentless pursuit I must have hit the right person at some point because at our last appointment the doc said something like "I'm being criticized for dropping the ball." It was pretty clear she didn't like to be thought of in that manner. But it was worth the hassle for us as we are finally able to meet her!

Wednesday is the fundraiser at Friendly's from 5:00 PM - 8:00 PM. Come see us and have dinner or ice cream. We are mostly looking forward to just being able to visit with you all. That reminds me, they suggested we have two people to sell 50/50 tickets for us (they provide the tickets). We will have a drawing at 6:30 PM and then again at 8:00 PM. So if you would like to be one of those people, please let me know!

Wednesday – Saturday, Frankie will be at Gilda's Club from 10:00 AM - 4:00 PM. All the kids there will either have cancer, or have someone in their family who does. I think it will be a great place for him to do some talking/thinking. He's been having some stomach issues, I think from some of the stress he feels.

Thanks for all of your love and support and we hope to see you soon!

So much to catch you all up on!

First let me say our kitty Oreo is now past the one month mark the vet gave him. Hurray for steroids! Actually, he seems to be gaining weight and has not seemed to decline, let's hope for more doctors being wrong ☺.

Secondly, we met on Tuesday with a woman Rose and her husband. She has been living with this diagnosis for two years (not three as I previously thought). They were a delightful couple and opened their home up to us. We will meet with them again down the road but got a great start. She started out at a lower stage than Tim. Initially she saw progress with chemo but eventually Roswell referred her to Hospice at which point she started treatments in Pittsburgh. Looking back, she wishes she had started out in Pittsburgh; they were not entirely impressed with their doctor at Roswell (which is the same doc we have). We have three more weeks to go before we start tests to show whether or not treatment is working for Tim, but we are absorbing all this information and keeping open minds about going elsewhere if it becomes necessary.

Last night we had an absolutely smashing time at Friendly's. We can't begin to thank you all enough for coming and being with us. First, let me say that the staff at Friendly's informed us this was the MOST SUCCESSFUL FUNDRAISER EVER for them. We had about 255 people come! Plus, they talked about how gracious and kind and patient everyone was when the waiting was so long. They said we were blessed to have so many wonderful people in our lives; of course we said we absolutely agreed!

Between the Friendly's money, donations from people who couldn't attend, and the very successful 50/50 tickets, the night far exceeded our expectations! You have all been so totally GENEROUS in so many ways, our words are inadequate to thank you. There have been so many extra expenses (like beds and stuff) and it seems like I am arguing about medical expenses more and more often lately. Your contributions are giving us a little breathing room this month, and we can't tell you how much it means to have less stress on us!

59

The most perfect ending to the night (which broke us down!) was when we were finally able to sit long enough and eat. That is when we found our very, very dear Mrs. Winters had secretly paid for our dinners. She was Frankie's kindergarten teacher and she is so dear to our hearts. She will have my head for telling everyone this story but I will take my punishment gracefully. We came home exhausted, mostly from being so darn thankful and amazed at all of you!

Today, Tim started another round of chemo. They figured out that his eyes have been feeling dry, which can be a side effect from the chemo. He thought perhaps that rather than feeling actual fatigue, maybe his eyes were tired from being dry. She started him on eye drops. His doctor told him — in a most cautious way — that his blood results may possibly indicate the chemo is helping... How about that for great news?

• Thursday, July 22, 2010 4:59 PM
Guestbook entry from Tim's family
Tim, Thanks for sharing this site with me. You are a very special person and you are in our prayers. If you need or want anything I'd be happy to help or talk or just listen if you want. I love you and believe in God being there for us all.

Ben is one of Tim's cousins who is the caretaker for his wife. She doesn't have that one diagnosis that explains everything, but multiple medical issues such as epilepsy, a blood disorder, and multiple strokes. He has been caring for her for over 20 years! I don't even have 20 weeks under my belt. I can't even fathom how a family handles these things for that long.

• Thursday, July 22, 2010 6:57 PM
Guestbook entry from Tim's family's friends
Dear Darcy and Tim, I am so ecstatic to hear that this has been a good week. Celebrate the blessings in your life! I will keep praying for positive test results. Tim, stay strong. Fondly.

• Thursday, July 29, 2010 4:08 PM, EDT

Tim attended a support group at Gilda's Club last night for the first time. This is what he had to say: "I met a group of seven people that had various forms of cancer, whose experiences humbled me. And some of whom had other life issues occurring in the midst of their cancer diagnosis that made me feel fortunate that I am surrounded by so many caring people.

"I found it nurturing. I found there was a lot to be gained from being there and striking up new friendships with people who are fighting for their lives. I found I had something to give. I am the youngest, and brought into the room with me, a high level of energy and enthusiasm and mental strength that all who saw it in me, got a great deal of enjoyment and inspiration. One guy had a six month old son that he couldn't imagine dying and leaving behind. That son is now 21 years old and 6'4" and is this man's pride and joy."

While this was obviously a great experience for Tim, he didn't make any more groups there. Gilda's Club is a beautiful resource, but it is not very conveniently located for us. When you are trying desperately to get through the days, even things like a longer drive become too much.

• Thursday, July 29, 2010 6:17 PM, EDT

Tim had chemo today and got more good news. Now I have the actual numbers in front of me. There is a number for "carbohydrate antigen nineteen" they call a "cancer marker." Normal level should be .0-35.0. His scores are still "abnormally high." HOWEVER... on June 8, his level was 12831.1, on July 1, it was 8510.1! I'm not great at math, but I think that is about a 30 percent reduction. On July 22, it was 6529.4, the latest data we have. Again, that is a significant drop on our books... almost 50 percent drop since this all started... Keep those prayers up!

• Tuesday, August 3, 2010 6:05 AM, EDT

Good morning! Today I take Tim for his CAT scan. This will be the big news as to whether the chemo is helping and how much. We probably won't get the results until next Thursday. If the blood

---

marker is any indication, we should be getting great results!

Add some prayers to your day for us. Tim's quality of life has been pretty down lately; he has had to come home from work more. When he's home he is sleeping a lot, but also just feels lousy most of the time. We are hoping this is some sort of cycle he will pass through, but of course we don't know; and there is so little I can do to comfort him when he's that ill...

We had our first "family meeting" to discuss how we are all doing here in our household. We plan to have them every other week. Frankie is also struggling; he feels homesick when he's away and wants to stay put more often. It is hard to juggle all of that when I have to work. Plus there are times I think it is better if he isn't home when his dad is so ill...

So pray for relief and mostly just wisdom to know how to handle all the challenges... we love you all!

Parenting in this situation has been... Well, uh... difficult. We have our older kids — Matthew age 23, Colin, age 26, and Emily age 29. Then there is Frankie, who is 7, going on 42. He is a very active and athletic kid who needs lots of activity and stimulation. So people have been great about having him over, taking him on outings, etc. It relieves me because he has my emotional makeup and notices everything. I see him worrying and being nervous about what is happening around him. But now he is telling me he is stressing out about being away too much. He needs to stay around home base more. I get it, I just wonder how I can possibly be the mom I want to be and be the wife and caretaker I want to be. I am very aware that the answer is I can't. I can't be all that I think I am capable of being. It's just not reasonable to expect of myself. I know that intellectually, but emotionally, it tears me up.

• Tuesday, August 3, 2010 6:07 AM
Guestbook entry from my supervisor
Darcy and Tim, Hang in there. You are on a roller coaster ride of healing. You have hit a low point but let your faith in the healing process help you climb back up to the next peak. I'm cheering you on... Love to all.

- **Tuesday, August 3, 2010 7:24 AM**
Guestbook entry from "Mom B"

Tim and Darcy, "We gain strength, and courage, and confidence by each experience in which we really stop to look fear in the face... we must do that which we think we cannot." - Eleanor Roosevelt. Love and prayers.

- **Tuesday, August 3, 2010 7:49 AM**
Guestbook entry from our church family

Good Morning, Darcy, You are doing such an incredible job balancing everything for your family! I so remember one of the times my mom was going through a terrible set back with her cancer (this was in 1996). She was in Roswell for three months, with infections, losing weight and my sisters and I were running back and forth daily, trying to juggle everything. When I was at work, I thought I should be at the hospital; of course when I would be at Roswell, I thought I should be with my husband or catching up with work... On and on it went for three months...

Then, the doctors decided to send her home once the infections went away and to "see what happens." Well, she rallied (actually for 11 more years!). My sisters and I look back at that time and know that it was God's grace and the love and concern of friends and family that helped give us the strength to keep going. Love to you and Tim.

- **Wednesday, August 4, 2010 7:59 AM, EDT**

Tim had his CAT scan yesterday; they also wanted to see him at the clinic after because he has been so sick. They decided his symptoms are probably chemo related, but are not bad enough to warrant lowering the chemo dose at this point. However, they do want to address the fatigue issue so they prescribed him Ritalin. That's what they usually use for ADHD, so people think it is a calming type drug. However, it is a stimulant, it helps the brain focus (which is why it is becoming a popular drug now for college students who want a "better edge"). So we'll see how that goes... thanks for those encouraging comments!

I'm not sure at what point we did this, but we ended up getting one of those pill boxes. It is the biggest kind, with places for pills morning, noon and night. I then put together a chart that explained which pills go in which box. Just keeping up with this alone feels overwhelming at times. There are so many things to stay on top of, and just when you think you have it down, something will change. Or many things will change. Tim used to handle his meds completely on his own, but it really is too much for one person to handle, especially if you are still attempting to live your life!

• **Wednesday, August 4, 2010 8:20 AM**
Guestbook entry from my colleague at church
"Strengthened with all might, according to his glorious power, unto all patience and longsuffering with joyfulness; Giving thanks unto the Father, which hath made us meet to be partakers of the inheritance of the saints in light: Who hath delivered us from the power of darkness, and hath translated us into the kingdom of his dear Son: In whom we have redemption through his blood, even the forgiveness of sins." (Colossians 1:11–14)

"Encouragement for today: In this world, we run short of patience and endurance. These are plentiful with God, however. We have an inheritance from Him — access to all His power, for He purchased our freedom Himself. For this we are to always thank the Father. We live now in the light, not in darkness. If anything is dark in your life, ask God to shed His light on it. Our heritage is light; we are no longer in the dark kingdom. Claim your inheritance of the light of life!"
— Diane Eble, author of Abundant Gifts: A Daybook of Grace-Filled Devotions

Chapter Eight:
What the Hell Just Happened?

I am having a lengthy conversation with Tim's doctor today (hopefully). I'm going to ask about test results in combination with the decline of his quality of life. He has now lost 33 lbs. and even finds it difficult to stand up sometimes!

On the positive side, we have finally booked a benefit for Tim! It will be Saturday, October 16th at the East Seneca fire department. "The Dustmen" will be playing. A very, very dear friend of Tim's is in the band. They are an Irish Celtic band so it promises to be a great evening.

Many of you have offered to help. I want to comprise a list of people who want to be on a "committee" of sorts. We will need people to help with food donations, coordinate theme baskets, handle raffle and 50/50 tickets, publicity, etc., etc., etc... So let me know ASAP if you are interested in this and we will all get together soon to discuss details. We love you so much... please keep the prayers coming!

So it has been another tough day here in the Thiel-Colvin household. I spoke with Tim's doctor this morning to alert her of Tim's physical symptoms, update prescriptions, etc.

My first journal entry was 7:32 AM this morning. The days are feeling like weeks now.

In spite of the blood cancer markers that were so positive, the CAT scan came back very disappointing. She said that is contradictory data she can't explain. The cancer has spread

> to his liver and stomach. Her plan is to stop this chemo regimen immediately and start him on a new one as quickly as possible. There is normally a two to three week wait, but we can't afford to do that.

What a ridiculously scary thing to hear. We can't afford two to three weeks? I can't even believe what I am hearing.

> Tim is very ill because of the cancer, not necessarily because of the chemo as we thought. His pancreatic ducts are now blocked (by what exactly I'm not sure) which explains why he is so sick. The pancreas is unable to function properly. She is treating this with an enzyme script whenever he eats anything. However, he has been too sick today to eat so he hasn't started taking them.

More drugs, different drugs. Can we even catch our breath?

> The explanation is this: when they give the initial prognosis of 12 to 14 months, chemo1 usually works for seven to nine months; they then usually start chemo2, which works for another four to five months. However, chemo1 just didn't work for Tim, so they want to start chemo2. When I pushed for prognosis, she said there is always the possibility that somehow he will react remarkably well to chemo2 and may still have that year. But there is no way to predict that and thus far he has not responded well to treatment.

BUT HE SEEMED TO BE DOING GREAT! He was tired but not even acting sick in other ways. His cancer blood marker was significantly down. He still works full-time for the most part. Someone please make sense of this for me!

> Statistics and treatment expectations are shaped like a bell curve. But Tim is not in the average, he is at the low end.

Isn't it bad enough to have a rare cancer? But then to have to be on the rare end of the stats? Is anything about this even remotely fair?

Most scary, is that she asked me if Tim "had" to work. I asked her why she would ask me that question. She said she believes she can try and control his symptoms now with medication, however, she can't say that by September. She thought he might want to reconsider work because if our family had any hopes or dreams, we might want to act on them NOW; so when your doctor says that... (Tim's response to that statement was "My dream was to live"...)

Wow, just let me sit with Tim's response for a moment. No, I can't. It is beyond heartbreaking.

Sorry to deliver such bad news. Please pray and pray and pray! There are so many, many decisions and choices to make; regarding getting a second opinion, treatment, working, etc., etc., etc. This is like when we first got the diagnosis. We are in a dizzy fog, not knowing what end is up, not even knowing what to make of it all. Tim took a lot of medication tonight, just to knock himself out. He went to bed saying "Tomorrow is another day" and that is true, hopefully, we will be rested and up to this new challenge.

We love you all.

• **Friday, August 6, 2010 9:18 PM**
Guestbook entry from our church family
Dear Darcy and Tim, My husband and I are praying that God helps you to know what's best to do.

• **Friday, August 6, 2010 10:16 PM**
Guestbook entry from our church family
Hi Darcy, Tim and Frankie, I will definitely be praying and praying. I am hoping and praying tomorrow will be a better day! Take good care of each other.

• **Saturday, August 7, 2010 10:57 AM**
Guestbook entry from our church family
Praying for God's strength, mercy, peace and grace to be with you all during this impossibly difficult time in your lives. Love and prayers wing your way.

In July, I had my 25th high school reunion. (Did I really say 25th?) It was very informal and out in the hicks where I grew up. Tim and I were able to go, although we didn't stay very long as Tim wasn't feeling great. But we got to see everyone again and we passed out flyers for the Friendly's fundraiser so everyone knew what was going on with us. This opened up yet another group of people who loved and supported us throughout our journey.

Oh my, oh my, oh my, oh my... where do I even start? First, my friend Ann, (from Chicago) is typing for me because Tim and I are at Roswell. Tim took Friday's news very hard and has been feeling very depressed since then. The weekend's ride was no longer a roller coaster, but more like those rides that drop you 20 stories all at once. Between the depression and the cancer progression, Tim's health deteriorated drastically. On Saturday, he developed several new symptoms including vomiting and hiccups. The hiccups were relentless. He was unable to eat more than a couple teaspoons of food, continued to grow weaker, could barely stand and turned grayish in color. He seemed to drift in and out of consciousness and was unable to hold a conversation. It was very, very scary. I finally called Roswell at 3:00 AM because the hiccups were so bad. They wanted him to go to an ER but he refused and said, "Go to the ER for hiccups? Are they crazy?" They prescribed medicine from the 24 hour pharmacy and we started to give him Gatorade and ginger ale.

Sunday morning I called our pastor's wife who is a Hospice nurse. Tim also has been exhibiting "altered mental status," which means sometimes he just doesn't make sense when he tries to talk. She gave us some advice regarding his medication and recommended another drug for hiccups because the first medicine was only minimally effective. Roswell agreed and gave him a new script which helped more but the hiccups did not totally go away. Our family, along with the nurse, came up with a plan, and to avoid going to a hospital Tim agreed to cooperate. We got him up, helped him shave, bathed him, cut his hair and got him dressed. He ate two teaspoons of pudding and two bites of banana. There is more to the story but I need to go talk with doctors now. More later.

(From Ann: They are ruling out bowel obstruction and Tim and Darcy are still at Roswell. Tim is coherent and trying to do sips of liquid and ice chips.)

Continued... sorry for the choppiness of the entries but I am writing between doctors' and nurses' visits... Where was I?

Sunday was Frankie's 8th birthday and we had a party for him which had been planned a while ago. We set up a lounge chair in the yard with pillows and Tim was able to come out long enough to hear us sing "Happy Birthday" and watch Frankie cut his cake. It was an improvement over the previous day but he still couldn't eat, struggled with hiccups, and continued vomiting. He eventually ate a couple of teaspoons of Jell-O but that was all he took the whole day. In the evening, our pastor's wife came over to look at him. She was somewhat encouraging as she felt he looked better than the way I described him on the phone but she agreed that he should go to Roswell first thing in the morning. At times, Tim appeared confused but he was able to reorient himself and she thought this was good. We struggled through another night at home.

Monday morning, after a few calls back and forth to Roswell, they told us to bring him in at 11:30 AM. He started having heartburn. He barely had a voice and it hurt to swallow. We had difficulty arousing him to get him to Roswell. I can't explain how difficult and scary this was for all of us! He literally had no quality of life or meaningful contact with us. The van ride to Roswell was a little tough as no matter how hard I tried, he was uncomfortable and felt jostled. We got him in a wheelchair and went to the blood lab. (This was a new experience for my sister, who went with us. It is very difficult to wait, side by side, with so many cancer patients.) From there we went to the clinic. Quite honestly, the nurses and doctors were shocked by Tim's appearance and rapid deterioration. The first person to see him was a representative from Palliative Care (i.e. Comfort Care). We had a lengthy conversation about Tim's medications and they decided to take him off everything to decrease his severe lethargy. They started him on Haldol to deal with his nausea, vomiting and hiccups and then Prilosec for his heart burn. The lab work showed dehydration. They started an IV to hydrate him and he seemed to get better initially. By the way, we couldn't get his weight as he was too weak to even stand.

Next, Dr. Hahn came in to see him, his primary physician at Roswell. We had a chance to ask her a boat load of questions but Tim tired of this. She and I stepped away and talked more. The cavity between the chest and legs is what we commonly refer to as the stomach. The cavity, but not the actual stomach, is cancer infested. The liver has cancer in and around it. She is unsure as to why the pancreatic ducts are blocked. They could do another stent if necessary but it would be unlikely that Tim could tolerate this procedure. All of these areas, plus the diaphragm, are not functioning properly due to the cancer agitating the nerves. Many of you have asked and YES, his lymph nodes do have cancer.

There's more but I haven't discussed the rest of the information with Tim yet so I'll update you all as soon as I can.

• **Tuesday, August 10, 2010 10:27 AM, EDT**

Continued... I just spoke with Tim and updated him so I feel comfortable giving you the rest of the information.

I had a lengthy conversation with Dr. Hahn about the chemo2 regimen. It has the same 70 percent chance at being effective as chemo1 did. However, it is much more toxic. The side effects would be worse. I asked her if he was likely to fit into that 70 percent group. She responded that, based on Tim's lack of responsiveness thus far, it would be unlikely that he would respond to this chemo treatment. However, it is all a moot point now because Tim needs to be much healthier before chemo is even an option. He needs to be functioning 'normally' at least 50 percent of the time to tolerate chemo at all. She seemed to feel that by the end of this week, we would have a good sense of whether his symptoms would improve or not. I also asked her how long we would have to wait before knowing if chemo was helping. She said that we could no longer rely on blood markers because they were not accurate for chemo1 (in Tim's case) but that they should be able to tell by symptom improvements quite quickly. I then spoke with her about my conversation with my pastor's wife, the Hospice nurse.

She has talked about research that indicates that patients who switch from curative care (chemo) to palliative care (comfort) tend to actually live longer. They are able to eat, sleep, be comfortable and have some quality to their life. Dr. Hahn said that she absolutely agreed.

Many of you have asked if getting a second opinion is an option. While we had discussed this previously, we have had little chance to discuss it again. It is highly unlikely at this point, however, that Tim could tolerate a trip to Cleveland.

The question of whether or not Tim will pursue chemo2, given the odds of its success, is uncertain. Again, this is a moot point now as he is not well enough to start it anyway. The one thing we know for sure is that Tim is stopping chemo1. This was obviously a difficult conversation to have with Dr. Hahn and just as difficult for me to inform Tim. I had to wait until he was coherent enough to understand the information. He is, of course, heartbroken.

Back to Monday, after Dr. Hahn and I finished talking, we returned to Tim to find him vomiting and having hiccups and pain again. His IV's were almost finished and she decided to do x-rays to see if there was anything else going on. We returned from x-ray and were getting ready to go home when Dr. Hahn returned and informed us that it appeared that Tim had a bowel obstruction. She wanted him hospitalized here at Roswell. She explained that the cancer activity seems to be causing kinks in his colon and that it would be better for him to be in the hospital until this was resolved and that she would send a surgeon in to assess the situation. My husband is stubborn and informed her that he would not be staying in the hospital unless I could sleep with him through the night. They pulled some strings, and I'll be damned, if they didn't get him a private room. He was transferred rather quickly to 7W, room 14. At this point, Dr. Hahn said Tim would either rally in the next 24 hours, or this might be it. The next couple of hours were a little difficult as my agitation and frustration increased.

We are really reasonable, if informed, but find it very difficult to be so when left in the dark. While the staff is very nice, once Tim was admitted to the hospital unit, they did not have the answers we wanted. Tim was given antibiotics and when I asked why, the nurse did not know. When I asked who ordered the antibiotics, the nurse did not know. When asked if a doctor was coming to see Tim, she did not know. When asked about the surgeon Dr. Hahn had requested, she had no knowledge of that. She said that Tim could no longer have ice chips but didn't know who ordered that or why. She asked me about his treatment earlier that day and had no information about what had happened in the clinic. She said "That was a different floor." I expressed concern about this and she sent me to the charge nurse. The charge nurse told me the name of the ordering nurse practitioner and informed me that she was the hospital nurse practitioner as I did not recognize her name. However, she did not know why antibiotics were ordered as Tim had no signs of infection. She said that sometimes they are ordered in preparation for a procedure. I again asked about the surgeon and she said that no surgeon would be in to see Tim, and that there was no doctor that would be in to see Tim, and that nothing would be done until 6:00 AM Tuesday morning.

I explained that this was <u>unacceptable,</u> as time is critical here, and that he was supposed to be treated through the night for his symptoms. She agreed to call the doctor on call in another part of the hospital. In the meantime, they paged a patient advocate at my request who did not respond to the page. About 9:45 PM, a doctor came and explained to me that the antibiotics were probably precautionary, that he couldn't have ice chips because of the possible bowel obstruction and that there would be no surgeon consult. At least we felt informed. Several minutes later the surgeon arrived, saying that Dr. Hahn had asked him to come.

It is my sense, that everyone here works very hard for you but unfortunately the left hand does not talk to the right hand. The surgeon explained that in his opinion, from the x-rays, the obstruction is not an actual blockage but a physiological response to all the cancer activity. The cancer movement is keeping all of those organs from working properly. He said Tim could absolutely have ice chips, as long as he wasn't vomiting.

He assured me that Tim would undergo no procedures and that we are strictly managing his symptoms. I asked him how we will know when Tim can go home. He said Tim needs to be able to tolerate food without vomiting.

Currently he has not vomited since 3:00 PM on Monday. We were hopeful this morning that Tim can have liquids but none of the staff here has any knowledge of the surgeon's visit to us. As of this moment, we have not seen any doctors this morning so we do not know what the plan is for today. We will update you as we can. This is really maddening, to say the very least.

At some point, some staff person made a suggestion that was invaluable — you should use it if you are ever in a hospital with someone. There is a large dry erase board in the hospital rooms here. I started writing down every single person's name that walked in the room, even if they were housekeeping. I wrote the time they came and exactly what they said. It was amazing that communication started to improve between staff and then with us almost immediately.

Keep us in your prayers, all your love and support is wonderful!

• Tuesday, August 10, 2010 11:10 PM, EDT

From Ann:
Tim is at Roswell again tonight. Darcy headed home to get a good night's sleep. Tim's brother Garrett was there visiting and Janet (Darcy's sister) was settling in as she is spending the night at Roswell to help Tim however he needs.

There is no concrete discharge date and while no one is pushing to take him home before he is ready, everyone seems to be working towards getting him home as soon as possible. He started clear liquids this afternoon and steroids to decrease inflammation of nerves and whatever else. No vomiting since Monday at 3:00 PM. The plan is to advance to other liquids after tomorrow morning's doctor visits. The hope is that he will keep fluids down and take in enough to be safe at home without IV's. He could go home with IV's but how much nicer to not have it? Don't know if they will require passing of gas or a bowel movement before discharge but they definitely want good bowel sounds before discharge! Goal: Get home ASAP... talk about chemo2 later.

Maybe he will go home tomorrow... maybe not, but he looks much better than he was this weekend. Had a lot of visitors today and was worn out but has his old sense of humor back.

(Remember to check CaringBridge and call friends for updates when you can... it really helps decrease the work on the Thiel/Colvin cell phones and at the Colvin's home.)

xoxoxoxo
Ann

On a side note, amidst all of this medical turmoil, we also met with the social worker. I mostly met with her by myself because Tim was out of it, and also because he didn't initially even know all the information about his prognosis. I needed time to talk to him but that hadn't happened before the social worker came. We are needing to look into disability benefits now. Tim suddenly seems unable to work, at least not at the pace he was. The whole process is ridiculously overwhelming and it's hard to even get approved. We've applied for some things on line but our Roswell contact should be able to help us navigate through the volumes of information we have to read and fill out. Of course, taking care of us financially seems unimportant compared to what we are dealing with physically. And yet, how do I not address this? I absolutely have to keep the roof over our heads. And more importantly, it seems to be Tim's main concern so I have to keep him not anxious about it. This is all too much for any human being to have to handle at the same time.

• Tuesday, August 10, 2010 9:50 AM
Guestbook entry from Tim's boss
You see the people you work with almost more than you do your own family so it's hard not to grow very attached. It may not be much but I have given a week of my sick time so hopefully you have one less thing to have to worry about. My wife and I are thinking and praying for you.

Tim's employer has been terribly supportive throughout this whole thing. Initially, they didn't penalize him any time off as long as he showed up for work. It didn't matter how long he stayed or if he had to leave, he got credit for the day. They couldn't do that forever, of course. The company actually set up a new policy so that employees could donate their vacation and sick time to another employee. It had never been done before, but Tim's situation inspired them to do so. We were very humbled by this, and so, so grateful. Providing for Frankie and me weighs heavy on Tim's mind so this helps tremendously. Several of Tim's colleagues donated their time to him. What a gift!

• **Tuesday, August 10, 2010 10:13 AM**
Guestbook entry from Tim's niece
Dear Uncle Tim and Aunt Darcy, I'm praying my heart out for you. I love you.

• **Tuesday, August 10, 2010 11:25 AM**
Guestbook entry from ?
Sounds like God is already working by sending the surgeon that others don't know about! Our prayers are with your family. We are also praying that the doctors, nurses, anyone connected with this case get the info from God as to what needs to be done. God performs miracles and we are expecting miracles! In Jesus name we pray, Amen.

We had no idea who this person was who signed our guestbook, but we were grateful for her supportive words anyway. After a few more entries, we ended up looking her up on the internet and discovered she lived far out west. Turns out she was a friend of one of my high school friends. Things like this would happen — people would hear about us from someone else and just lend us their support. And with the availability of the internet, you can meet people across the country. It is truly amazing!

• **Tuesday, August 10, 2010 3:03 PM**
Guestbook entry from my college friend
Hi Darcy, I read every entry you submit. My heart is so heavy for you. I am praying for you and Tim and Frankie. What a difficult time for all. It is my hope that you feel the prayers surrounding you. I am sorry for what you are going through and pray there will be some light today to brighten your outlook.

• **Tuesday, August 10, 2010 7:14 PM**
Guestbook entry from Tim's niece
I love ya Uncle Tim! I'm praying 4 u.

• **Tuesday, August 10, 2010 11:18 PM**
Guestbook entry from my cousin
Love cures people — both the ones who give it and the ones
who receive it. I am praying for you.

Chapter Nine:
What the Hell Just Happened? (Again!)

• Wednesday, August 11, 2010 8:22 AM, EDT

Well, I don't know what my sister did last night but Tim woke up feeling much better. I haven't gotten to the hospital yet but Tim called and said that he wants to come home. He wants to go back to work a couple of days a week and wants to start mowing the lawn again. They are going to have to hospitalize me next! (I'm only half kidding.)

And oh yea... now he wants an MP3 player. This is technology neither one of us knows anything about. (I know, we are way behind the times.) I'll get him whatever he wants, so all you experts out there just tell me the make and model and where to get it.

Will check-in later.

The news has been so bleak and scary, I wanted to get this entry off as quickly as possible. I was so shocked when Tim was talking coherently on the phone. It was like a miracle.

• Wednesday, August 11, 2010 7:39 AM
Guestbook entry from my high school friend
Hallelujah! Jumping for joy today here in Rochester! Still praying, too ☺. Love and hugs.

• Wednesday, August 11, 2010 7:49 AM
Guestbook entry from my Dad's friend
Hi Tim, Darcy and sons, I think of you all day long, and hope Tim has been free of pain and discomfort. You are all special to me as are all of your dad's family.

• Wednesday, August 11, 2010 10:37 AM
Guestbook entry from my high school friend
Hi Darcy, It was great seeing you and Tim last month at the reunion. With all that you have to deal with, I was SO pleasantly surprised to see you there! After reading just a few of your guestbook entries, I can see that you have so much support from your friends and families. Well, I always say that you get back what you give! Make sure you ask for help when you need it, that's what we are all here for and sometimes people just don't know HOW they can be of help to you. Ok?

• Wednesday, August 11, 2010 7:01 PM
Guestbook entry from Tim's colleague
Wish I could say something to help, wish I could do something to help. Please tell Tim I wish him well, and I will be by to see him as soon as I am able.

• Wednesday, August 11, 2010 9:23 PM
Guestbook entry from Tim's former in-laws
Uncle Tim, Aunt Darcy, Emily, Colin, Matthew, and Frankie, I just want to let you know that I am praying for you and thank you for sharing your journey of faith, love, and hope.

• Wednesday, August 11, 2010 11:54 PM
Guestbook entry from Tim's former in-laws
Uncle Tim, Aunt Darcy, Emily, Colin, Matthew, and Frankie, I can't imagine how hard this must be for each and every one of you. It is brave and incredible to keep an online journal of your daily personal activities, struggles, and feelings.

• Thursday, August 12, 2010 11:17 AM, EDT

I am very exhausted and bleary eyed, but I want to try and make an entry before I pass out!

So... after the usual hospital communication issues, we were finally able to get Tim discharged from Roswell last evening. There were several issues with his medication scripts to square away but we are able to keep up what Roswell had going. I strongly suspect the key ingredient to all this was the steroids. That is what has turned our cat around and once that was started for Tim, he really took off also; yeah for steroids!

He is a bit manic now! He is eating normal foods (for the first time since his diagnosis) in smaller amounts. He could hardly sleep last night. He is running around washing dishes, doing laundry, skimming the pool, complaining about how things have gotten run down since he stopped participating in the household. He has gained seven pounds... CRAZY! Is this a miracle?

He's pretty cute; the steroids also make him very emotional, so he cries all the time... good crying. We all crack up, someone asks him a simple question like "What would you like to eat?" and then we see it in his eyes — uh oh, he's going to cry again ☺.

I wish I had more time because there is so, so, so much to explain. When I walked in yesterday morning and saw him standing and walking around the room, I was caught off guard. I was overwhelmed with crying, like a major meltdown. (Of course Tim was crying too because he always cries now.) I was like, "You almost died and now you want to mow the lawn? I don't know what to do with you!" Maybe a few more expletives than that... I was relieved and rejoicing eventually, but initially I was just like a wet noodle. I remembered that I know this about myself — when it is really, really dark, I usually stay very strong. The second Tim improved, my body and emotions just fell apart and collapsed. I don't know if that is the opposite of most people or not, but it feels so weird to me. In the middle of the crisis, I hold my head up and push through. When I felt like I should be crying with happiness I folded into a pile of mush.

Anyhow, I'm being kicked off the computer. Later I will write more about the medical plans for the future and also about what you all need to know about how to proceed from here. Maybe I can even get Tim to write.

• Thursday, August 12, 2010 11:24 AM
Guestbook entry from my Dad's friend
Steroids are GREAT! So glad he and you are doing better. What a rollercoaster. Hope you enjoy the salad if dad remembers to bring it!

• Thursday, August 12, 2010 11:52 AM
Guestbook entry from my friend in Chicago
Today is Good - Carpe Diem!

• Thursday, August 12, 2010 7:31 PM
Guestbook entry from our church family
Hi Darcy, You actually made me laugh when you said, "You almost died and now you want to mow the lawn." I guess that sense of humor, or whatever it is that helps one cope when times seem totally out of control, is God's way of helping...

So glad Tim is home. I agree that steroids are a miracle drug and can recall my mom talking a blue streak (more than usual, which is where my sisters and I get it from) when she would take them. I am keeping my fingers crossed that you and your family can enjoy an UNEVENTFUL weekend!

• Saturday, August 14, 2010 10:43 AM, EDT

Ok... in spite of how bad it is for the environment, I've decided to use paper products in the kitchen to help cut down on the clean-up time around here. So forgive us Mother Earth!

I feel I have so very much to tell you all, but am under time pressure and constraints. I apologize if things are disjointed, don't make sense, or if I leave gaps. Please ask any questions you might have as I'm aware I'm overtired and too time constrained.

SO... Tim has been home since Wednesday night. Get this — he went to work for a half day on Friday! He's a kook! Anyhow, his new plan is to work Tuesdays, Wednesdays, and Thursdays, then have a four day weekend. He will stretch out his vacation/sick time that way, plus his company is allowing people to donate their time to him. Thank you to all you amazing co-workers! Also, he does not have to work a full day on those days, but can just do what he can. He also has the option to work at home from a computer if that becomes helpful. We can't say enough about how caring and supportive his company has been throughout this process!

Tim is on steroids. We have been informed and are fully aware, that these help tremendously. The caution is that people can easily trick themselves into thinking their medical condition is also improving. This is not the case. Tim's prognosis has not changed.

When discussing the chemo option with his doctor, it has become clear that the treatment would be very toxic to him. In addition, the chances of that chemo even helping at all are very slim based on where he falls on the effectiveness curve. Given all of that information, he has decided not to pursue treatment at this time.

If he should ever choose to do so, insurance will pay for a second opinion. I have gathered as many records as I can. Cleveland Clinic is ranked third in the nation for cancer hospitals (Roswell is 33) and that would be where we would do a chart review. HOWEVER...Tim is not choosing that option at this time. If he ever changes his mind, things will be in place to do so quickly.

Secondly, there has been much research done (especially recently) on palliative care (hospice, a.k.a. comfort care). Patients often end up living longer when they switch from curative care (like Roswell, chemo, etc.) to comfort care. People are able to eat and sleep more comfortably, have a much higher quality of life, and end up living longer. With all that information given, Tim has chosen to sign on with Hospice.

Hospice will continue to work with Dr. Hahn, who is fully in agreement with this decision and has agreed to cooperate with them. A nurse will come to our house once a week, but they are on call 24 hours a day, seven days a week. All his medicines will go thru them and be delivered to our house from now on. They also have a chaplain who happens to be from our church who is on his care team (we are care team number five). A social worker also checks on us weekly. She is setting up someone to work with Frankie at least until school starts and he can be back in his normal environment. (Last night I had a difficult conversation with him about how daddy has the kind of cancer where he will NOT get better. This seems very hard for him to understand. He is also worried now about dying when he is 50 because his paternal grandparents did and now his dad is dying at age 48. I am working on this with him.)

We have about an $1100 deductible for Hospice left (it was $3600); but we decided to go with them (even though a lesser known option was available with no deductible). It is all about who you know and we have MANY significant contacts at Hospice that we can rely on if we ever need to.

As I said about the steroids, right now Tim is functioning very well. He is alert, coherent, and mobile. However, the doctor made it very clear that we have no idea how long that will last. Or he could also drop like last weekend and hit those extremes a few more times. SHE HAS STRONGLY ENCOURAGED THAT ANYONE WHO WANTS/NEEDS TO HAVE MEANINGFUL CONTACT WITH TIM SHOULD DO SO NOW — sooner than later. If you want to visit, have special alone time, have that burning conversation... please don't have any regrets; contact me and we will set some time up for you. Don't hesitate, use this time he is feeling well very wisely.

We are actually going to my sister's campsite for the day. We may even sleep over if he is feeling well enough to do so. We will be back Sunday afternoon.

Thanks for all that love and support!

Camping is one of the things that we have grown to love as a family. We started out in tents. That first year I swear there was a thunderstorm every single time we went camping. So it lost its luster quickly when we had to come home and clean mud off everything we owned. We were able to get a little pop up camper that we love. We prefer to go in May and September/October because during our short summer months we love to stay put right at our pool. My sister has a permanent camp site about an hour away so every year our whole family spends a weekend together there. This year, it would end up just being a day. In spite of having a good time, Tim wasn't feeling well and we had to come home. But we did have a lovely day.

• Saturday, August 14, 2010 3:09 PM
Guestbook entry from my friend
Hi Tim and Darcy, Sounds like you two have really spent some tough time making some very tough decisions. You two are

83

both such a blessing. Thank you for sharing your journey with us. I know that personally it has helped me tremendously. I am going to have my husband read it also. Hopefully it will give him some guidance too. You are in my thoughts and prayers.

Jill's husband also has cancer. His prognosis is not good either. He has been dealing with it longer than Tim has, but they haven't been exposed to the resources and support we have, in order to be more prepared. We are truly grateful if our events end up being helpful to someone else. It is one of those sweet gifts alongside our bitter truth that we are blessed to be aware of.

> • **Monday, August 16, 2010 8:18 AM**
> **Guestbook entry from Mom B**
> Tim and Darcy, I have just read your most recent entry and I believe that all of the choices that have been made are the best ones. I admire both of you for all of your courage on this journey. My thoughts and prayers are with you.

> • **Tuesday, August 17, 2010 9:48 AM**
> **Guestbook entry from my family**
> Hi Tim and Darcy, You are all in our thoughts and prayers and have been for a long time. You have been through a whole lot of stuff since the family reunion. Please know how sorry we are and how much we love you guys. Please let the Lord comfort and give you peace even in the worst of times. I know it doesn't seem as if He is with you but I hope you know that He has never left your side. I also pray that you guys are able to talk to a good Christian counselor/mentor. Believe it or not prayer does help. Our prayers are not always answered in the way that we wish but they are answered. Our girls from Washington are here and will be going back in a week. Perhaps we can meet on Monday the day they go home.

You know, it's been interesting for us. Tim and I have definitely gone through our own spiritual journeys in our lives, complete with plenty of "mad at God" and "Why have You abandoned me?" phases. But for whatever reason, we just haven't gone there this time. Neither one of us has. We have truly felt God beside us every step of the way. Our sense is that God is grieving and suffering with us, and wishing like we are that someone would find a cure for cancer. I think the biggest factor is the love and support we have been surrounded with. It's hard to stay full of self-pity when so many others sacrificially give to you over and over again.

As for counseling? Now that's our forte. Besides it being my profession, I am also a personal lifetime fan. I can't imagine a time when I would ever think I had life figured out enough that it wouldn't be helpful to have a third party to kick ideas around with. Tim and I have been with a counselor for the entire ten years of our relationship. Our kids have gone with us too at times. Now Tim is not a fan. He has made it clear for the whole ten years that he would just as soon not go. He is still saying that today. However, it is quite obvious he has been grateful to have Scott in our lives. Scott has actually come to the house to do sessions when Tim hasn't been feeling well. Plus, in many of those private conversations we have shared with each other, he's said a lot of "You know you've been right about this stuff all along" kind of statements. Neither of us can fathom going through what we are going through without our trusted counselor, Scott.

• Thursday, August 19, 2010 4:23 PM, EDT

As usual, a lot of life has been lived before I've had a chance to update this journal. First, we had to put our very beloved cat Oreo down last night. As the vet told me, steroids are like a miracle drug. The catch is they only work for a short period of time. It was a very emotional time for all of us as we said goodbye and then buried him in the backyard next to our other cat Pooh Puddin'. And thanks to Dr. Peters and her staff who were so kind and gentle with us during this difficult ordeal! And thanks to my understanding clients who once again arrived for their session only to be sent home...

Losing a beloved pet is usually traumatic for most people, but the parallel in our lives is almost too much for us to comprehend. We were given the same speech about steroids for Tim.

Tim worked seven hours on Tuesday, six hours on Wednesday. He came home and talked about the jobs he was able to get out the door because he was there. He is energized by feeling like a vital part of his workplace — and he is!

Today he came home though at 10:00 AM. He is frustrated with his medications. We spoke to Beth, our Hospice nurse, and she is already scheduled to come tomorrow morning at 11:00 AM. But there is one medication we were already trying to wean Tim off of which contributes to his lethargy. We are also seeing if he can go back on the Ritalin to boost his energy; she also gently reminded us that expecting Tim will bounce back to his old self before the hospitalization symptoms, is probably not realistic; his initial bounce back was very fast and sudden, which was great — but the reality is that overall there will be a decline in his health; she suggested he reconsider his work schedule as it may be too much for him; sooooooo... he's thinking about all of that but is just trying to rest when he can for now.

I am overwhelmed once again with all there is to do. And again, people's generosity and kindness to us is equally overwhelming! We are trying to take things a day, more like a minute at a time. But the task for Tim to maintain his health is a great one. The task for me to manage all that needs to be managed is also a great one...

So keep praying for us and sending all that love and positive energy. We suck up every drop of it ☺.

Love you all...

The day that I brought Oreo home to be buried in our backyard, I was greeted by some of Tim's family I had never met before. I may have mentioned before that one of the gifts we receive that is a direct result of the cancer diagnosis, is the reuniting of people that were long disconnected. After apologizing for meeting them while we were all a sobbing mess, there was a lovely talk on the gazebo. I was able to witness bridges being rebuilt while things that were long overdue were said. It turned out Mark lived a couple of blocks from Hospice. Down the road he was one of the most helpful of Tim's family members, coming to check on Tim daily, sometimes even several times a day. The bitter-sweet. Bury our pet, introduce loving people into our lives. All within minutes.

• Friday, August 20, 2010 8:21 AM
Guestbook entry from Tim's childhood friend
Tim, I want you to know that my wife and I pray for you all the time. We also have you on several prayer chains at several churches (you can never have enough people praying for you).

It was very nice seeing you when Jim and I visited you in Buffalo. You have a wonderful family and I know that they are a great help and support to you. I'm very sorry to hear that the meds aren't helping you and that you've had to cut down on your work schedule.

I know how you feel as I have been taken off work completely since June (my heart is too weak the doctor said). I know that when things get tough, having a good attitude makes a huge difference and trying to concentrate on the blessings we have rather than on what we are losing makes us appreciate each precious day that the Lord has blessed us with.

It was beyond our comprehension how people who were afflicted with their own life traumas, could still find energy to support us. I know we feel like we can barely get up and get back to bed every day, yet some of these people faced tough circumstances AND gave to others. Humbling.

• Saturday, August 21, 2010 2:57 PM, EDT

Hello to everyone!

Today is going to be a big "how you can help" email. Tim's daughter Emily and her son Parker are flying in shortly today to visit for a couple of days. We're excited of course!

Anyhow, a bunch of stuff is coming up. First, Tim wants to make his own picture board of his life. As we have time, he will be selecting files off our computer. We don't have any actual prints made up so if anyone (or a few of you) wants to volunteer, we could email you the shots we need. You could print them for us. If a couple of you share this task, it shouldn't be overwhelming.

Secondly, we had our first meeting to start planning Tim's benefit in October. Now THAT was overwhelming. It is like planning a wedding but only having six weeks to do it. The ways you can help are absolutely endless. It will be held Saturday, October 16th at East Seneca fire hall, from 2:00 PM – 9:00 PM.

Send me an email and let me know what you are interested in. We are scheduling people in two to three hour time slots to help with the following-
1- keeping up with food being out
2- setting up
3- cleaning up
4- selling tickets at the door
5- selling raffle tickets for baskets
6- selling 50/50 split tickets

In preparation, we have a form we are working on for basket donations. If you are interested in making one to raffle, or know of any contacts of local businesses, there is a form to fill out. From what I understand, this is one of the most crucial parts to the day.

The other big thing is donations to the actual event. We are looking for as much to be donated as possible. This includes chips and other snack foods, sheet pizzas, and desserts. There will also be beer, wine and soda. If you know ANYONE at all or are willing to make phone calls for us, please let me know.

I feel way out of my league here. The "committee" is dedicated and experienced and they assure me they know how to run these things and will help to make it manageable. Your help is key to making this a success!

So, we know you have given and given to us, and now we are again asking for more from you... please let me know how and if you are able to assist us.

We love you!

The benefit is supposed to be first and foremost a fundraiser. Even though Tim has life insurance, the financial pressures ahead are never far from our minds. And Tim is particularly concerned about making sure Frankie and I are left in good condition. But the more we plan this thing, the clearer it is to me that it is about something much bigger than fundraising. It is about me giving my husband his day. It is about Tim knowing what it feels like to be the guest of honor and be surrounded by hundreds of people. It is about him saying goodbye to them and them saying goodbye back. It's going to be a celebration, one hell of a party. It's the epitome of the bitter-sweet life we are leading.

• Tuesday, August 24, 2010 8:16 AM
Guestbook entry from my family

Hi guys, The family would like to do a gift basket and my husband and I can help with making sure the food is out. Hope to see you soon. Love you guys.

• Tuesday, August 24, 2010 9:40 AM
Guestbook entry from my client

Darcy and family, I will be happy to donate four baskets (toy oriented) for the benefit. It was great to see you both out last weekend.

• Wednesday, August 25, 2010 10:43 AM, EDT

Regarding the benefit - we have a flyer designed in color. We are looking for someone to search for a donation for printing or if anyone has access to a color printer or color copier at work who could print them for us. Please let me know as soon as you are able.

We also need to print the sheet raffle tickets for basket donations. If anyone has a contact for that let us know that as well.

Thanks to all!

• Wednesday, August 25, 2010 7:27 PM
Guestbook entry from our church family

Hi Darcy, We can get the sheet tickets reasonably. The cost is about $30. How about if I purchase them as a donation to the cause?

- **Thursday, August 26, 2010 12:39 AM**
Guestbook entry from Tim's family's friend
Dear Tim, Darcy and family, Steroids can definitely be a double edge sword... they improve your daily life but watch out for the long term. My husband and I always felt we would take all the good days we could get... and thank God for the steroids! So I am happy to hear they are giving you some relief.

I am excited to hear about your benefit. Please count me in for a basket to raffle. In the meantime, enjoy these last days of summer. Know that you continue to be in my prayers for courage, strength, and peace.

- **Thursday, August 26, 2010 11:48 AM**
Guestbook entry from our new cyber friend
Prayers are with all that are connected to Tim and family. We can't be there as we are not close enough to help do the physical things, but we are keeping the prayers going. God knows what needs to be done, so we will leave it up to Him. God bless.

- **Thursday, August 26, 2010 4:28 PM**
Guestbook entry from Tim's colleague
Hi Tim and Darcy, I have just finished reading all the previous messages sent to both of you and all of the journal entries - here I sit with tears in my eyes at all you have had to endure. Life is not fair and the older I get the more I believe that.

Tim helped me often at work. I was always bugging him for help with various problems. He is truly one of the good guys — always helpful and pleasant — the type of person you want and need in your "work family." These are the people I miss. I retired almost five years ago. Tim, you are so lucky to have the huge support system around you! I look forward to seeing you at the October benefit.

- **Friday, August 27, 2010 5:27 PM, EDT**

I just put this massive, long update on here and I somehow lost it. So let me try again...

There is so much to update you on but I've not had the time to keep up as I'd like to. We have been visiting funeral homes and cemeteries and let me tell you, it exhausts us on every level...

Big news is that we have changed the benefit date. Quite honestly, we are very worried about Tim's health and where he might be by mid-October. So we have moved it up to Friday, September 24th, 5:00 PM - 10:00 PM. I know this may be inconvenient for many of you but please understand where our priorities must be at this point...

If you check the photo album you will find the flyers for the event. Feel free to print them, email, and Facebook them. We will have copies printed if you need a stack of them.

Also, the benefit committee is working hard and has also tried to relieve some of the stress on our household. Shirley is the overall director (pays to have a friend who is a professional event planner!). Below are listed the areas of ways you can help. Please try to contact the appropriate person directly for areas you are interested in.

Also, we could use stamps for mailing out tickets. If you want to donate a book of stamps or something, that will help keep our expenses down as well.

This is much less detailed than my first attempt but please keep forgiving us. Our lives are so crazy and exhausting. We truly are doing the best we can!

Making the decision to switch the date of the benefit was tough. People were already working hard but this would make the deadline even sooner. But it became more and more clear to me that this wasn't just about raising money, it was a celebration for Tim. And I wasn't sure by October 16th he would be feeling well enough to really enjoy it and soak it all in. It wasn't that I was trying to be pessimistic. It was that all too familiar impossible catch 22-trying to be positive and healing minded with being realistic and accepting.

• Saturday, August 28, 2010 9:45 AM
Guestbook entry from my high school friend

Darcy, I was very taken in by Tim's story and the struggles that you and your family are faced with. I know it's been many, many years since our paths have crossed but I felt it necessary to reach out to you and let you know that my thoughts and prayers are with you and your family during this very difficult time. May the Lord give you the strength, courage and comfort needed to get through. Love and God bless.

• Thursday, September 2, 2010 9:12 AM
Guestbook entry from our cyber friend

Sending prayers your way for Tim as well as everyone connected to him. Everyone needs to have the strength that God can give so I will be asking for that. May the angels wrap you in their arms and give the comfort that is needed. God performs miracles when we expect them and we are expecting them. Amen.

Chapter Ten:
A Screeching Halt

Jeeeeeeeepers... so much happens in a day, much less a week; so I'll try to give you the quick synopsis.

Saturday and Sunday, Frankie had a nasty fever, he recovered well in a day or so, but the three of us lost a couple of night's sleep, poor kid!

Tim had a great weekend and on Monday decided to go back to work another day a week (this makes four) because he seems to be on an upswing. (Yeah for Tim!)

Then by Tuesday, I had the nasty fever, bad night, and wicked chills. Wednesday morning, I got up to take a call, ended up passing out and hitting my head on the floor. (Yes, there is still a very sore spot on my head.) My nurse neighbor insisted on my going to the ER to be checked.

So we had to smile about the role reversal for us. This time Tim was the driver and I was the one moaning in the car. Turns out, they say it was a "blessing" that I fainted and wacked my head. Otherwise, I would not have gone to the hospital and found out that I have silent pneumonia... so how's that for terrible timing?

They could not seem to get my blood pressure back up to normal but sent me home anyway after three liters of IV's. (BP still low...) It took another 24 hours for the fever to completely break. Now I just have a headache and throat issues but I'm VERY grateful that I am not shaking from head to toe with chills! (It is truly amazing how your perspective changes — bump on the head becomes a blessing, and so does a headache when it is not a chill ache.) So I'm on antibiotics and am ordered to have lots of rest for weeks and low stress (this isn't something you recover quickly from... don't they know how busy I am?) and I find I have to rest. I can be up briefly but then tire very quickly.

Bad timing for the benefit, as things are in a frenzy of activity, but our capable committee is dedicated and they keep reminding me over and over that Tim and I are not supposed to be worried about it anyhow. They are handling it! Thanks to all you amazing supporters... what would we do without you?

This was a big, huge wake up call for me. As if it wasn't enough for us to juggle all we had to emotionally with staying positive and yet realistic every day, now I had to face my own limitations. I had worn my body out. For good reasons, but I was worn out none the less. My body was forcing me to slow down. I was literally unable to get up at times so I had no choice.

> • **Friday, September 3, 2010 7:29 AM**
> **Guestbook entry from my Dad's friend**
> Hey guys, Darcy, please take care of yourself! Dad is keeping me posted, but you're the healthy one! Everyone I talk to tells me they wish the very best to you two. Love you guys!
>
> • **Friday, September 3, 2010 9:54 AM**
> **Guestbook entry from our cyber friend**
> God is trying to tell you that you need to slow down and let some others help you! Yes, guess it was a blessing to have a bump on the head. Am saying prayers for anyone connected to you all that everything can go in order and all fall into place for the benefit! The angels are everywhere around you, so just relax a bit and not stress out! Let the prayers work. Amen.

So the vast majority of people responded to us in this supportive manner. But there were some tough points along the way. For the most part, people are who they are, and relationships are what they are. When significant crisis arises, sometimes people and relationships band together in ways they couldn't imagine to battle whatever is facing them. But sometimes, bad dynamics only get worse, and then you sit and wonder why you thought they could get better with all that extra stress around?

My family is ridiculously supportive. They are located anywhere from

50-80 minutes away, but time and time again would drop anything to come and be here whenever they could. My sister actually took an unpaid leave of absence from work on two different occasions to come and help take care of Tim. But not all families function that way and I would dare say that most probably do not. It's just the way it is for whatever reason. All families have their strengths and weaknesses.

I felt like I wasn't a big hit with some of Tim's family when we first met. That's all I will say about that. But the night I got home from the hospital after my fall, an already tentative relationship blew up on a phone call. In some respects it was a big misunderstanding, but in other ways I guess it was inevitable. I don't ever intentionally hurt anyone, but I am human, and therefore thoroughly flawed. I had made an implication that offended someone, even though I didn't intend to. It was over the level of involvement some of Tim's family had in our lives, and more specifically around the benefit.

Some of them weren't fond of computers, which isn't a problem in and of itself, but it was our only means of communication. I guess I should say it was the only one we could keep up with, and even that was difficult sometimes. There was just no way to make calls to individual people and family members to let them know what was going on. And because they weren't around us on a daily basis, they had no idea the chaos and nightmare we lived in. It was like a big line of falling dominoes. If you weren't here, you didn't know how terribly hard our life was. And if you didn't check your computer, you couldn't be updated that way either. So there were big gaps of information missing.

So in the conversation, I was not implying that Tim's family wasn't helping us. We were entirely grateful for any amount of interest anyone paid us. But sometimes they just truly had no idea how complicated things were and didn't have the big picture in mind like other people did because they didn't have all the information. The call ended badly and I cried for almost an hour. The upshot was that I was officially "cut off" and was "done with" by some of Tim's family. So much for resting at home, cutting back on stress, and trying desperately to get better.

Those who know me, know I work very hard at being truthful, but always and always tactful. My husband was dying, I was under incredible strain, and I was extremely physically ill. Yet somehow, none of that mattered, and whatever crime I had committed, was completely unforgiveable, even under the circumstances.

95

As I went to sleep that night, I had to tally the day under the "bitter" side. However, when I awoke about 4:00 AM and discovered Tim wasn't in bed, I realized there was more life to be lived. I found him in the living room. He had been awake all night. He was very disturbed by what happened between his family and me and was unable to shake it. We have gone through lots of transformation over the last couple of months, and Tim had just experienced another big one. He saw me enter the room and said "Darcy, God has given me an epiphany tonight." Oh boy, his tone was serious. He went on to talk about how the last ten years had been shaky between his wife and his family and how that had caused him distress over the years because he loves all of us. He said that he had been evaluating his life with me throughout the night and wanted me to know that he had consistently asked me to "be the bigger person" whenever conflict had occurred between me and his family. While in and of itself, that isn't a bad thing, he said he saw now how that had just served to set precedent with his family. His dislike of confrontation usually caused him to avoid it, so that is what we generally tried to do. But he felt completely resolved that God had spoken to him during the night and said that he must set things right before he died. He was being given a chance to do the "right thing."

As I listened, I asked him what that meant exactly. He said he wanted to write a couple of his family members and let them know how he felt. He didn't feel like I had always been treated well and he needed to let them know how much he loved and respected me, and that he demanded others treat me that way as well. It was time to set the record straight and be the supportive husband he needed to be. It was no secret that Tim and I had a pretty rocky marriage at times and have been in counseling throughout its entirety. But that didn't mean he didn't love me deeply and the events of the last couple of months had certainly changed our lives and relationship completely. Again, he made it clear that this message came directly from God. I listened, quite honestly, in shock. I suggested that he try to get some sleep and when he was rested if he still wanted to send the letter, then maybe he should.

Too late. He had already written and sent it. Email, immediate, no taking it back. I was incredulous. It was a beautiful letter, but I couldn't believe he sent it. In my heart, I knew that I was moved beyond belief. I knew that I had longed for a decade to have him defend my honor. But was this the right time? All I can say is that it must have been, because Tim was utterly convinced without a shadow of a doubt that this was meant to be. He believed with all his heart that God had given him an opportunity to right some wrongs that had been done. And once again, I was humbled. While I had gone to bed with a terribly hurt heart, there was a gift in the center of it. I felt a closeness to my husband that I had never felt before. We had a bond of loyalty and love that can only come through adversity. It was a true transformation, born only from being willing to take the bad with the good.

I didn't realize the collateral damage though, at first. I didn't know yet the night before was the last true night of sleep Tim would ever have. When he stayed up all night, he got off his sleep cycle. He never got it back after that, and that would have devastating effects on his overall ability to fight his disease. But again, the bitter and sweet, hand in hand.

Chapter Eleven:
Back to Work,
Whatever That Ends Up Being

• Tuesday, September 7, 2010 3:17 PM, EDT

First day of second grade for Frankie! Dad had suggested Tim go in late to work and get Frankie on the bus (first time!) so he did! We were thrilled ☺. Frankie insisted on wearing his suit... is he cute or what?

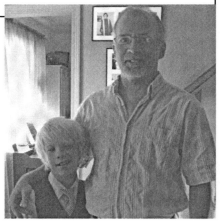

This was one of those things that made me smile. Prior to this year, I couldn't really get Tim to do things like go in late to work so he could see Frankie off on his first day of school. Those kinds of things were always "mom's job." Not this year. This year Tim takes every opportunity he can to make memories with us. It's a lovely thing.

• Tuesday, September 7, 2010 3:05 PM
Guestbook entry from my Dad's friend

Frankie is a cutie. Only grandpa wants him to have a haircut! Hope all is well lately, and the two of you are doing ok!

• Tuesday, September 7, 2010 3:25 PM
Guestbook entry from Tim's friend

Your son is adorable and I wish him lots of fun in second grade while he is learning. Hope that Tim is well. Dads usually aren't the ones taking pictures on the first day. That was awesome for all of you.

Another new thing for us is walking. Tim always said "I don't walk." Period. I'm definitely not a big exercise person, but I always thought if I had someone to walk with, that wouldn't be so bad. After ten years, Tim finally relented and said we could get a dog. But he reminded me again, that "I don't walk, not even dogs." But having Taffy forced me to get out and walk every day. Somehow amidst all of our changes, Tim decided to have a go at walking. He then decided he even liked it! He can't believe how nice the little parks are near us, and is even more surprised at how friendly people are. I keep telling him it's dog people — they tend to be friendly. So we would walk Taffy and chit chat with people and know it was good for our souls. Eventually, we started taking the wheelchair for Tim as his physical energy would die out before his emotional energy did. He kept the leash in his hands and I pushed the chair. It took us awhile to get the rhythm down but we eventually did.

Then I got pneumonia. And our brief routine got changed again. Now, we do our usual thing half way around, but then we switch. I sit in the wheelchair and hold the leash and Tim pushes us around. I think Tim is pretty proud of taking care of me while I take care of him. And I have to admit, it feels good to sit in my exhausted state and have him tend to me. I'm sure we are an interesting site to onlookers, but we don't care. We love this new ritual!

• **Saturday, September 11, 2010 10:03 AM, EDT**

Hey everyone...

Small update — we saw the Hospice nurse yesterday. My blood pressure is up to 100 now which is a positive improvement. Tim's vitals remain perfect ☺. Because his insides are not functioning properly, his stomach is bloating some. This is then pushing on the liver and other organs so he is experiencing some pressure in those areas. However, they will just keep an eye on it at this point because he has no other symptoms (like terrible pain, etc.). It is better not to mess with anything (like a drainage procedure) until it becomes necessary.

So we're moving along a day at a time. Hope all of you are doing well as you start the new school year and get back into routines, etc. We love you!

• **Saturday, September 11, 2010 6:33 PM**
Guestbook entry from our church family
Hi Tim and Darcy, I am so glad that we finally met today. I felt a real connection to both of you and I also knew I was in the presence of a deep love. Hope the rest of your day was peaceful.

Molly was someone that attended the same church as we did, but we had never met. She contacted me because she belonged to a charitable organization that was having a benefit in October. They like to have two people or organizations to divide their proceeds between and we were selected! We were surprised and thrilled, to say the least.

I am a list person, someone who needs a system to accomplish what I do. I know I'm a little OCD-like, but I figure it's not such a bad vice to have if I'm going to have one. When Frankie is in school, there are always many things to handle each day. That is not unique to me or us, but every once in a while, the absurdity of my list hits me like a brick, smack in the middle of my forehead.

Hmmm... Make Frankie's lunch. Pick up the house. Run errands. Pick out a cemetery plot with my terminally ill husband. Make phone calls. And we would just go down the list each day and do the best we could. But then I would get stopped dead in my tracks and think, does anyone realize that this list is crazy? Crazy?

Talking about cemetery plots also made for some uncomfortable conversation. My parents bought double plots before my mom died so that was all settled for them. We hadn't considered this and we had to make a similar decision. I didn't really want to get a plot for myself, not knowing where my life would be heading. I didn't want to hurt Tim either though. I have not decided yet, but I think I would prefer to be cremated anyway. Turns out that most plots you can have one additional cremation burial on top of a casket. That made us both feel better. We aren't going to add my name to his head stone, but at least we know I can be with him if that seems the best down the road.

So one day we went to look at cemeteries. Neither of our parents had plots that were close by. That was important to Tim because he felt bad he didn't get to see his parents' cemetery very often because it was a long hike. He wanted his kids to be able to visit often. We finally decided on a lovely place within walking distance of the church. Tim said he could just see Frankie and me walking there after church services and it brought him comfort. Of course, it was the usual bittersweet experience. Bitter to be picking out a place to be buried in at 48 years old. But Tim somehow made it enjoyable.

We were looking at plots with the caretaker and Tim laid down on the ground. He said that if he was going to spend eternity there, he had to know if it felt right! The caretaker assured us he had seen crazier things than that. Tim told me that he wanted to be buried with a word-find book and pencil in his casket. I said "Really? And what do you think you will do with that?" He thought for a moment and said "Good point, it will be dark. And I suppose it would be a bad idea to light a match in there. Can you put a flashlight in there too?" So of course I promised him. Word-find book, pencil, and flashlight. Just in case he wakes up and doesn't want to be bored. I love that man.

• Tuesday, September 14, 2010 5:42 AM, EDT

Hello to everyone!

The benefit committee has asked me to post some specific needs as this website is the quickest way to reach the most people. The committee people are absolutely knocking themselves out and dedicating lots of time to make this a big success for Tim. It is a celebration!

First, they are trying to sell as many tickets in advance as possible rather than buying them at the door. That way we have a much more accurate number for having enough food, etc. You can call the contacts for that, or we have tickets here as well.

If you have a box of old picture frames, we could use some simple 8 x 10 size for putting raffle gift certificates together. It is helpful to have any basket donations as soon as possible. It is a lot of work for Shirley to put everything together and label them so the less that has to be done last minute the better.

We have had excellent food donations, but still need vegetable and fruit trays.

We could use all paper products — styrofoam cups, small plates, large plates, napkins, and forks.

There has been a shotgun donated ($500-$600 value!). There are $10 raffle tickets available for anyone interested. Shirley and I have tickets for that.

After the meeting on Wednesday, there will be one more update regarding what kind of volunteers we still need for the night of the benefit. There is GREAT entertainment lined up. You won't be disappointed!

Thanks, as always, for all your love and support. This is all so exciting and Tim is really looking forward to seeing all of you. Emily, Spencer and Parker are driving in this week for a few days and we can't wait to see them.

Stay tuned ☺.

I have decided to make Tim a surprise gift. His colleagues from Texas sent him a DVD of all of them saying hello, showing him the plant, etc. It gave me an idea of making a video for him. I enlisted his help and told him we are doing it for all our guests at the benefit, so he prepared a welcome speech as well as a thank you speech. What he doesn't know, is that in between I am going to video people from various aspects of his life, giving them a chance to say something special to him. With Tim not working as many hours these days, this is proving quite challenging for me to sneak around to tape. Plus, I'm doing groups of people so that is tough to organize in and of itself. Part of me thinks I'm crazy with everything else going on, but it has become my mission. This party is the surprise 50th birthday party I may not be able to throw him. It comes from the depths of my heart and I want to shower him with love.

Especially difficult is taping Tim's co-workers. I need to tape most things when he is at work. But of course I can't tape his work friends when he is at work, so that presents a problem. I'm not sure how I finally pulled it off, but I did get there one day. As I was saying goodbye to them, one of his neighbors asked if he could talk to me. A couple of others gathered around so I was sensing he was going to ask me something that many of them were wondering. He asked me if I could help them understand where Tim was really at. They were all reading our site and knew that the prognosis was grim. And yet Tim was there, day after day, still "taking stairs two at a time." He was productive and pleasant. It just didn't make sense to them. I felt such compassion for them. And I knew I couldn't really explain it either but I did my best. I told him that Tim and I found it confusing too. All we knew, was that the steroids were like a miracle drug. They made him feel and function much better, but we had been warned not to be fooled by them. They are telling us he is very sick, and his prognosis is not good. So that's the best we can understand it. They shook their heads in understanding. I think that it was what they had already thought, but just needed to be sure they weren't missing something.

Before I left the building, the General Manager showed me to his office. We sat down and he closed the door. We had a similar conversation. As best he could, through his tears, he told me what an invaluable employee Tim was. He explained that he would take a thousand Tims and run his entire company with them if he could. He assured me he was entirely sincere and wasn't just saying nice things because Tim was sick. But then he also awkwardly asked me why he was still at work. As much as he was desperately needed there, he said he wanted to shake Tim and tell him to go home and be with his family. I again felt such compassion for him. I opened up to him and said that when this first started, I struggled with resenting how much time Tim spent at work. I was hurt because I couldn't believe that was his priority. And yet with time, I had come to see it much, much differently. I told him that Tim felt confident and alive when he was at work. He was battling a disease that was taking his life and he had no control over it whatsoever. When he walked through the doors at work, he was in control, doing things and accomplishing things, and making a difference in the world. And most importantly, he was earning a living. That was monumental to him — and that was out of love for Frankie and me and wanting to be our provider. So I assured him that while it may seem crazy on the surface, Tim was exactly where he wanted to be as long as he was physically and mentally able — at work. We both seemed comforted by this conversation.

Frankie's school has been amazing. The principal and social worker do an incredible job. His kindergarten teacher was beyond delightful. At the end of first grade was when Tim first was diagnosed. His teacher was supportive and alert to Frankie's questions and needs. Now he is starting second grade. This year's teacher is no different. I will consider her a dear friend by the time this school year is out. She talked with me about writing this entry, agonizing over what to say and even how to sign her name. She need not have worried. She was another angel God sent to us.

Sunday, September 19, 2010

My minister went on Sabbatical June 1st and will return on October 1st. While he was gone, people volunteered to preach to fill in. I had volunteered for today as I have preached a few other times in my life. (I graduated with a Bachelor's Degree from Moody Bible Institute.) At the time I signed up, I had no idea Tim was sick or how our lives would change.

Most of the staff I work with at church are extremely supportive, especially because Reverend Miller has been gone for most of Tim's illness. Several times I was approached about being let out of this responsibility to preach that I had signed up for. I knew people thought I was crazy for still doing it, and I thought perhaps I was too. But I had this burning desire to see this through. I truly felt like the message in my heart had to be spoken or I would burst. I know God's Spirit works that way sometimes so I decided to trust it, in spite of my busy schedule.

It was a day to remember, and a service people would talk about for months. One of my best friends in the whole world, Summer, and I ran the service. Tim was there and many of our family. The sermon was about the depth of God's love. I started out talking about our church family and asked people to stand that had helped us in various ways — putting up the fence, making prayer shawls, bringing meals, shopping for us, praying for us... Of course by the end, almost the entire church was standing. It was quite a testimony for the way God was using them to minister to us.

The basic premise of the sermon was that if God had a wallet, my (your) picture would be in it. I showed several pictures of Frankie on the power point screen to demonstrate how gushy parents are when they brag about their children. Then I drew a powerful conclusion that God finds us delightful, in spite of knowing our darkest secrets. Later in the service, I sang a solo about trusting God as the "Shepherd of My Heart." Later, Summer prayed for our family.

I believe what moved people was the genuine and open spirit that we were there with. Everyone in that building knew about our situation. Everyone knew Tim was sitting there. Everyone knew that Tim was dying. Tim knew that he was dying. We laid it out for everyone to see, and then we still could testify to God's amazing love for us and the trust we had in God's guidance and transforming power in our lives. No mistake — we were coming from a deep, dark, struggling place and could still love the God of our faith. It was very moving to say the least, and like I said, people talked about it for months. I knew in my heart that I did the right thing. It was a message that just had to be given.

• Sunday, September 26, 2010 9:49 AM, EDT

My goodness, it has been ages since I have been able to update this. I apologize. I know you understand our lives are crazy, but I really wish I could do things more consistently. I will try to remember the details as best as I can.

First, let me update you on Tim's health issues. On Wednesday, he had his usual weekly visit from Beth, our Hospice nurse, his vitals were normal and things remained status quo. By the way, Tim had increased his work to four days a week, and most of those are full seven to eight hour days. He had also gained eight pounds in one week, but the bloating is still not problematic.

Wednesday night, about 3:00 AM, Tim awakened me because he was having difficulty breathing. He could breathe, but only on a shallow level. He complained of "pressure" in his upper chest. He was unable to move in either direction in bed, but had to remain perfectly straight and flat. Of course, he didn't allow me to call Hospice until the morning...

I spoke with a couple of Hospice nurses Thursday morning. Their thought was that with the weight gain and his bloated stomach, the fluid was beginning to push his lungs up, causing him difficulty with breathing. A fluid drain would be a Roswell procedure so they would set things up with them.

Late Thursday morning when we spoke to Roswell, they said they couldn't get him in until Friday morning at 11:15 AM. I was going to push to get him in right away but Tim was rather fearful of the procedure and didn't want to go anyhow. He felt he could live with the discomfort another day although he didn't move much from the bed or couch all day.

Thursday night was another restless one for both of us as Tim's symptoms increased. We went in to Roswell Friday morning and were sent to ultrasound which is where they do the drains. They use the images to navigate where they go, however, much to everyone's great surprise, the ultrasound showed very little fluid. It did not warrant a drainage procedure at all. In fact, there wasn't even enough fluid to allow such a procedure. The doctor did an ultrasound on his back and again saw little fluid, however, they were suspicious of pneumonia (boy did I feel bad!). He called Dr. Hahn's clinic and we were sent over there.

There he saw our PA from the old days. She sent him for a chest x-ray that came back negative also. They did an EKG which also came back normal. They gave him an IV push and pain meds. They asked him to start taking his anxiety medicine again and gave him an 800 mg script for Motrin for inflammation. We were there until 3:30 PM (yes, the day of the benefit)!

When we got home I spoke with Hospice Beth again. She was as shocked as we were, as all indications led to fluid. Sooooo... the good news was, all the tests were negative, the bad news was, we don't know what is going on. Anxiety/stress may certainly explain shortness of breath to some degree, but that does not explain the weight gain and bloating... So next week we have to decide where to go from here, basically whether we will pursue more answers, or continue to treat the symptoms only.

Tim was able to attend the benefit for a while; he was in bed all day Saturday but is feeling a bit better this morning. We are planning to go away for the night to Niagara on the Lake for some much needed rest...

When we return I will send an update on the benefit (which by the way was beyond incredible!). Thanks for your patience!

Again, confusing and scary. You think you have a relatively good idea of what is going on. Then you go in and you are flabbergasted. What in the hell could be going on if that wasn't fluid? And we are sitting there, surrounded with love and family, but having no idea what we are facing. The benefit was in a couple of hours too. Were we even going to make it there?

Chapter Twelve:
The Benefit

Ah, THE BENEFIT. What a loaded event. Weeks and weeks of fun,
upset, stress, and excitement all packed into one night. Before I show
the journal entry I wrote
about it, there is much
to say that did not get
"published" out there.

As I mentioned, Tim was
able to come for awhile.
The highlight was when his
best friend from Michigan
came and surprised him.
Tim tuckered out though
and our friend Summer took

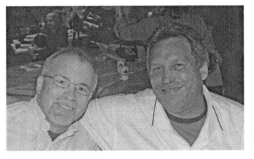

"Coop" and Jim

him home and kept him company. I ended up having a bit more to
drink than I planned on. But I have to admit it felt really, really good.
I danced, visited with people, and got a little silly. There was a clown
there that did face painting. I had him paint "I LOVE" on one cheek
and "TIM" on the other. I thought I was pretty adorable until I went to
the bathroom later. I was sweating buckets and the paint had dripped
down my face, making me look like something out of a really cheap
horror film. Boy, did I wash that off fast!

Throughout the weeks of preparation, I had some conflicts with a couple
of friends of mine. Their version of the story is completely different I
am sure, but for me it was all pretty confusing. I know one of them

felt like I was being a "control freak" and should have not even been involved in the details. I felt like the benefit was an incredibly large but personal gift to my husband and I wanted a certain atmosphere there. It was like someone that plans a baby or wedding shower in your honor but then doesn't ask you what you want so you can enjoy it. It's all very awkward when people give of themselves ceaselessly to you, and you feel like you can't say anything about how it's going without sounding ungrateful. Afterward, several of my closest family and friends processed it all with me. It was hard on them too. They heard things get said about me that were unkind, and even untrue. While the friendships survived, they have never been the same since.

On a good note, we had about 180 baskets that were donated! It was kind of crazy. There were tables of people who won several items, and then people who won nothing at all. There were some larger ticket items that had separate raffle tickets. Tim's family won a $200 set of tools. Unfortunately, someone stole it. We had heard about things like that happening at benefits and it's hard to believe but it really does happen. Some smaller baskets were taken too, but the big one was very disappointing. The harder part though, was the upset that was caused. The gentleman who had won the stuff was very angry. I don't think he was as upset about losing the items as he was that someone dishonored his family in that way. The entire situation with Tim being ill is intense enough, but then add this and it was just too much for him. I heard stories about it for several weeks. He apologized later about it and all was forgiven, given the circumstances.

The politics around a benefit are as difficult as a wedding is. Everyone wants things to be perfect and everyone works hard. But then there are funky dynamics that go along with it. One of Tim's family members talked at length with one of my kids that night. There was a big emphasis on how all those people at the benefit were there mostly because of the efforts he put into it. He did work hard, but he had no idea just how many people contributed to its' success, and for weeks longer than he even knew about it. But I also got a little insight into one of the reasons some of Tim's family struggles with me. The complaint was "That Darcy, she always has to try and fix things." I thought about that one a lot. I decided that if that is the worst thing that someone can say about me, I am doing pretty well with my life. I mean, it still hurts that people talk about me (especially to my children), but really, I guess that's not so bad. Lots of times I *can* fix things. I've certainly been a fierce advocate fighting for my husband's life and he is nothing but deeply grateful for it.

Remember the family member that was angry and "finished" with me? She was at the benefit too. She worked her butt off. I heard nothing but how hard she worked from start to finish. She was amazing. I give her credit. In spite of any feelings she had toward me, she never let it interfere with how much she loved Tim. And he was what mattered now.

The DVD was amazing. Maybe mostly to just Tim and me but that is all that truly matters I guess. We sat in the front row and watched it. I was extremely frustrated because people talked through it. But with over 400 people there, I guess that should be expected. Let me tell you what it consisted of.

It opened with Tim introducing himself. He is sitting in front of our computer. "Hello everyone, I'm Tim Colvin. Some of you know me as 'Coop'. I'd like to tell everyone why we are holding this benefit tonight. Prior to April of this year, our family had a typical life in progress — work, school, home. I, myself am an engineer. I did my engineering work, worked side jobs, came home, cut lawn, did lengthy to-do lists. Tried to be a husband and a father. Typical life, like everyone else. Unfortunately, the type of life that swallows people up and time speeds along. In April, I had some tightness near my gallbladder. It was initially diagnosed as gallstones, which happens to a million Americans every year. So I went in, and after the surgery was over, I was told by the surgeon that I had stage IV gallbladder cancer. While that was a punch in the gut, it made me the epitome of how something so wrong could happen so randomly to a guy. How clever of a cancer that it had given me no symptoms, it just (snap of his fingers) came upon me.

"So we're holding the benefit because I am only 48 and I've got another 15 years before I retire. So that's 15 years of lost income or basically 14 or 13 because I am trying to manage to make it a little longer here. One thing this illness has given me however, is the ability to appreciate life on every level imaginable. Just like those mushy emails that people get, I now enjoy every minute of life. For instance, I had no idea that I had come to know so many people in my lifetime. You go through life without counting really. God has blessed me with each and every one of you. I am honored that at some point in my life, our lives have crossed paths, either for a day, a week, a month, or a year. The truth is, each one of those days, months or years has been the best of my life...

"In the background I was listening to a song called 'You Make Me Feel

Good' which is a Zombies B side that a band played when I used to go to their gigs. I think it's appropriate because all of you tonight have made me feel good by coming out tonight and showing your support by coming to this benefit. So thank you all for coming and I hope you enjoy the rest of the festivities. Love you all and thanks again."

Tim wrote that himself, and that sums up so much of how he views his life. The life expectancy for his diagnosis has not exceeded two years that we know of, but he truly plans to beat those odds. My emotions flood as I listen. He truly means every word of it, his new found appreciation for life flowing every day.

The next clip was entitled Tim's 'former in-laws, but always family.' Tim was married for 16 years to Sheila and had three children with her. Divorces are often ugly, but we had worked very hard in the last few years to develop a civil relationship with Tim's former wife. He always had a good relationship with Sheila's family and they did what they could to be supportive during this time. So the whole group of them got together for me and told an amusing story about how Tim mooned some poor old lady in the picture window during a garage sale. Yep, Tim's sense of humor.

Next up were his colleagues. They said they think of Tim like a hummingbird because he is always buzzing around the office. What a perfect description of him. I have always said he only has two speeds, zero and 100. His colleague said in the video that he only has one speed and it's "very fast." I can just visualize him at work, going a mile a minute. Hummingbird. Good symbol. There were also some jokes about what a hearty eater he is. So true.

Tim's older brother Garrett talked about how he was charged with "watching his brother" as they were growing up. There was footage from his family at his brother's cottage. They all have a sense of humor. For as long as I've known Tim, they have gotten together regularly for "brother's night out," although brother was extended to any family member. They have a great time together.

My family shots were next. No doubt that Tim was considered family from the very beginning. He was famous for his sense of humor and always shocking everyone with the unexpected. They also talked about the many times that Tim was willing to offer a helping hand with whatever project they were working on. We were the recipients of my family's help many more times than we ever helped them. That's just the way our family is. Truly we are there for each other. But nothing could compare to how they have stood by us as we battle this illness. Tim's best friend Jim and his wife were next. He told a story about them when they were kids and how they burned their fort down by accident. They were grounded for months! Next was Tim's younger brother. He spoke with emotion about times that Tim protected him and took care of him throughout his life. He said Tim would always be his big brother, no matter how much taller Roger might get. Through obviously genuine tears, he called Tim his lifetime hero.

The next section was Tim's four children. They shyly talked about their dad and how he was able to fix things in their lives, no matter what the problem. Our youngest, Frankie, mentioned hockey a couple of times. They have a lifetime of memories around hockey games and stories. And in spite of feeling a bit awkward having their lives telecast for all to see, they told their dad they loved him.

Tim's big brother Garrett came back on. He was commenting on their day at the cottage together, but it fit perfectly for the benefit as well. "This has been a wonderful day. It's been a lot of fun. Good food, good beer, a lot of laughs... Tim has been the star of the show. That's why everybody came... It's a special day that we will always remember. But keep in mind, we are looking forward to more days, just like this. We are certainly not done partying or celebrating. We look forward to the next time, whatever that means, for however long that means."

The last section was me. I found a copy of our wedding vows, which we had written ourselves. I thought they were perfect still, ten years later so I decided to record them as an ending to the DVD. "Hi Tim, remember these words. I love you. We had a very magical beginning and then life has kept us busy ever since. When I stop to think of your many qualities, it brings tears to my eyes. You are romantic, poetic, sensitive, motivated, and energetic beyond the call of duty. I promise to be faithful to you. I promise to try and be the very best partner I can be, in every facet of what that means — spiritually, socially, financially, emotionally, and physically. It is my personal and heartfelt goal to hear you say at the end of your life, that two hearts are better than one. That our lives were qualitatively better beyond compare because of uniting with each other. This is my commitment to you."

Tim's friend took my video camera and recorded us watching the DVD together at the benefit. It is some of the most precious footage I have of us. I worked so hard on this surprise for him, and I knew he was deeply moved. It is a memory that will last a lifetime.

• Tuesday, September 28, 2010 9:05 AM, EDT

There's still so much to update you all on so I will do my best...

First, we cannot possibly begin to find the words to thank everyone for the absolutely amazing benefit on Friday. So many of you worked tirelessly, (Ok, I know you were tired... more like exhausted!) and gave of your time over and over and over again. It was a monumental effort and we thank each one of you for all you did to pull it off.

Second, thanks to all of you who attended, donated, invited friends, etc. We had over 350 tickets turned in at the door! So that number does not include kids or people who trickled in or volunteered to help. Estimates have been between 400-500! The greatest part is, the fire hall people told us they haven't had an event that big since they joined — not even for weddings! What a testimony to how much you all love Tim... we are overwhelmed, not even sure how to let it all soak in.

The financial support far exceeded our expectations as well. We have been so deeply moved by the generosity we have seen repeatedly, and the stories about how people have donated who have no idea who we are! Make no mistake — THERE IS MUCH GOOD IN THE WORLD — MUCH, MUCH, MUCH!! So when you have a down day, or someone does something not so lovely, keep the big picture in mind!

If I was told that this book could only be one sentence long, I think this would be the one I would choose. It is the lesson that is engrained most deeply in us, even while surrounded in the knowledge that cancer is a hideous disease. ***Make no mistake — THERE IS MUCH GOOD IN THE WORLD — MUCH, MUCH, MUCH!!***

Our time at Niagara on the Lake was brief, but amazing. We decided the phrase of the day was "bitter-sweet." We have never stayed at such a beautiful place. Our room was exquisite (did I spell that right?). The bed was sooooooo comfy. We even had a fireplace in the room which we kept going through the evening. First thing we did was notice the large jet tub in the bathroom — room enough for two! So we climbed into the warm, soothing waters, breathed a very deep sigh and snuggled in. We looked at each other and quietly started to weep. Words weren't necessary, but we agreed that it was ok to bathe in each other's tears. We were so relaxed, relieved, exhausted, treasuring each other's company, but knowing these moments are numbered.

After that, we went down to dinner. Thank goodness our waitress was lovely. We didn't know what the heck we were doing. We didn't even understand half the descriptions of the food so she helped us out. The food was fabulous and we were stuffed to the gills! About midway through dinner, an elderly couple sat at the table next to us. We discovered it was their 68th wedding anniversary! Again, we looked at each other and began to weep quietly. It became obvious what we needed to do... When we left, we let the waitress know we wanted their bill to be sent to our room. It was a precious connection we felt with them, and somehow wanted to celebrate our own 68th anniversary through them. We know you aren't supposed to tell anyone when you do something nice for someone, but it was such a spiritual and intense moment for us, we wanted to share it with you. It was an opportunity directly from God.

On Monday, we walked a bit around the village but Tim was not feeling well. We used the wheelchair but decided to go home early and cancel our massages. It was brief, but it was perfect, a highlight of our lives together ☺.

Tim stayed home from work again today. He's not in any pain, just having a very low energy level. He's hoping to return tomorrow.

Thanks again for all your love and sharing our journey with us!

• **Tuesday, September 28, 2010 2:31 PM**
Guestbook entry from Tim's friend
Sounds like a wonderful time for you both. So glad you got to spend some quality time together even though it was short. Thinking about you daily and saying a little prayer to keep you strong. You both are amazing!

• Tuesday, September 28, 2010 2:55 PM
Guestbook entry from my high school friend's parents
I am so deeply moved from reading each of your entries... your's and Tim's journey triggers all of my emotions... treasure each day and each moment... remember you are both loved and prayed for by many persons... let our strength be yours at this time...

Chapter Thirteen:
Extreme Roller Coasters

On Monday night, Colin brought home "Louie," yet another addition to our family ☺. He is very beautiful but Taffy keeps her in the basement most of the time. He totally brightened Frankie's spirits! I was sitting on the floor when we let her out of the carrier. He came over, crawled on my lap and started purring. I knew he would fit in just fine here.

Tim has worked partial days Wednesday and Thursday. I have a call into the doctors just because I am curious about what the possible causes are for his symptoms now that we know it is not fluids... keep praying ☺.

As usual, this update is long overdue... life can happen so quickly around here and before I know it there is so much information that I haven't been able to get to you! Thanks for your patience...

Tim had a pretty rough weekend. He was very uncomfortable in any position he tried to sit, stand or lay in. He began to take pain medication for the first time. His breathing was very labored also. By Sunday, I was VERY concerned and called Hospice back again. A nurse came out and that was tremendously helpful. Today, our regular nurse Beth came out as well and was also tremendously helpful. So here is the best I can do to summarize.

They took Tim off of the pain meds he was on and put him on methadone twice a day (morning and night). This is a narcotic that has less side effects than others. (Tim was complaining about feeling exhausted and out of it, while wanting to jump out of his skin at the same time.) In between doses, he has a morphine equivalent for break through pain. He has not needed to use that since the first night.

He was given foam wedges for sitting which has helped him a lot with comfort also. In addition, they gave us a foam insert for his bed which should also help relieve the pressure he feels from his enlarged belly.

Beth was just here last Wednesday and she was a bit surprised at Tim's sudden turn around. On Wednesday, his stomach was enlarged but soft, today it is hard throughout the whole area. On Wednesday, he had no swelling at all in his legs, now he is swollen from his ankles up to his knees. Apparently this is very rapid for fluid gain.

One side of his lungs is now quieter than before. His blood pressure and heart rate were both higher than usual. All of these things are strong indicators of fluid. Deciding whether to attempt another drain at Roswell is based on two factors — breathing and pain. The new meds should control both, if they are unable to, a drain would be considered. However, it is not preferred because often fluid is drained only to return in 24-48 hours.

She also noticed his coloring was off. She "couldn't quite put her finger on it" because he is not pale, but the yellow tone is not the typical color associated with jaundice either. (I agreed when he was jaundiced it was different.) His color is noticeably "off."

Tim also can only eat very small quantities. There is little room left in his belly for his stomach so it makes sense that he eats less. While he tries to keep liquids coming, she said we shouldn't "push" them either. I expressed my concern over the August episode when he was critically ill due to dehydration. She explained that these changes are "expected" rather than "acute" which relieved some panic I was feeling.

He has also experienced a lot of confusion and at times even delusions. This may be due to the pain medication, but it may be due to disease progression. The next week will be critical. The hope is that his body will adjust to the meds and he will be pain free but without that loopy kind of thing. But again, we will have to wait and see.

She has put an order in for a massage therapist to help relieve some of his back aches and also for compression stockings. Yeah, you got to love those, right Karen? (Karen is my friend that has to wear them.)

So what this all means, is another major change in our lives here. Because of his confusion, Tim needs 24 hour care now, not a nurse, but he should not be left alone. I also now manage his medication completely as he has been confused about when he has taken pills or forgotten them. We also have to keep the medication stored away because of the narcotics. Tim could accidentally overdose when in a confused state.

He is now pain free, but sleeps most of the time. It is hard for him to have any meaningful conversation. Please pray especially this part will improve by the end of the week.

So, we will need you now more than ever, I am canceling everything I possibly can but still have work obligations. If you would like to be on my call list to come and sit with Tim, that would be very appreciated. Often times I need help spur of the moment. Colin is an immense help but he is also working and helping tremendously with Frankie.

As always, thanks for your love and support!

Even as I read this over again, I am shocked at the turnaround of events. Every one of these paragraphs seems like a sudden, drastic change. That feels crazy to say when you've been fighting stage IV cancer for four months. And yet it seems drastic and like it occurred almost overnight. What just happened? What just happened??

• Tuesday, October 5, 2010 6:31 PM
Guestbook entry from Tim's friend
Sending lots of prayers your way to help you be strong at this time. I admire both of you for your courage.

• Wednesday, October 6, 2010 10:20 AM, EDT

Beth (Hospice nurse) is coming again today, they sent

compression stockings yesterday so he's been wearing those. They seem to help once you finally get them on ☺.

Tim was a little better yesterday — could walk a little without dizziness. Our minister came by and he was able to converse about 15 minutes before falling asleep (a big improvement).

The nights are brutal though; it has been several nights in a row now that Tim hasn't slept through the night. He gets up several times for different reasons. Last night was especially tough. I finally got up with him at 3:00 AM and laid on the couch. Pretty soon Frankie joined us so I think we are pretty much exhausted. Tim sleeps most of the day on and off, but I think he needs to do that in addition to a solid night's sleep. I'm wiped out but am not able to nap through the day so I start to see stars after awhile ☺.

We will see what Beth says today. I know she wanted to put him on a night med but Tim had it before and didn't like it. Perhaps today we can talk him into it...

Thanks for all that support ☺.

• Wednesday, October 6, 2010 5:41 PM
Guestbook entry from my supervisor
Hi Darcy, Sounds like things are rough. Please call me if you just want to talk...Thinking of you and your family often... Do you need any help with your clients? Love ya.

Ah, my clients. That is a tough one. I am still thinking that I need to be available for Tim for at least several months. How do I take time off now when I need to figure this out longer term? I don't have the kind of job where someone else can step in for a shift. My job is based on the relationships that I have built, but also must maintain. Sometimes I think I am crazy to try and work. And yet in a very real way, my office is where I regain my sanity. In that room, my life makes more sense. In that room, I am more confident and feel like I can see where my efforts make a difference. I can close the door and pretend the other part of my world doesn't exist for awhile. So when is the right time to take a leave of absence? This is a decision I struggle with daily.

So much life gets lived every moment it seems...

Don't know where to start. Tim continues to be wakeful throughout the night. It is so hard to explain. Throughout most of the day and night, he dozes on and off, sometimes for 30 seconds at a time. He usually goes from the bed to the couch. He may settle in bed, look sound asleep, and by the time I walk to the next room he is up again.

Sometimes he is aware of his surroundings while other times he is confused. He is frustrated because he can no longer manipulate a computer mouse (although he will sit in the computer chair and promptly fall asleep sitting up). He also says he is unable to turn a light switch on or off.

Yesterday Colin was mowing the lawn. I didn't even hear Tim go out the door but he went outside and promptly tripped over the hose and fell. I heard him yell and went running. Colin said it wasn't a bad fall but he was a bit muddy. Thank God he didn't injure himself, but safety is becoming more and more of an issue.

Last night, around midnight he got up a couple times and tried to get ice and water from the fridge door. He just watched the ice spill over and over then the same thing happened with the water. Then he repeated the behavior ten minutes later. It is so hard for me to know how to handle some of these things. I don't want to insult him or dampen his spirits by encouraging him not to do ANYTHING, but his perception and balance is so off. I don't think it is very safe for him to do anything. Yet literally all night he gets up and down, walking aimlessly. You will swear he's in a deep sleep and suddenly he's standing next to you.

About 10:30 PM last night, I went to get my neighbor who is a nurse. I was concerned about Tim's breathing. She said it was like sleep apnea. He would take two breaths and then there would be a pause. She demonstrated the type of breathing that I needed to be worried about so I knew what to look for.

At 2:00 AM, I called Hospice anyway. I had the nurse listen over the phone. She said he was pausing up to 15 seconds between breaths. She called the doctor and we got one of his meds increased. (Tim will not take one of the meds they want him to so this is one he is amenable to.)

The regular nurse is coming back today (that makes four visits this week for Hospice nurses). She may want to recommend Tim go to the in-patient Hospice unit. Tim is very opposed to this. They would like to get his sleeping and agitation under control. I want him here at home just like he wants to be here at home, at the same time, I'm scared to death. He fell yesterday and I was here! I woke up at 2:00 AM one night and saw him standing on a step ladder in the bedroom trying to change the smoke detector batteries.

I'm VERY sleep deprived now, so... I will keep in touch with everyone as things unfold. I've got overnight coverage tonight because if I don't get some sleep I think I will completely crash. It is hard to ask someone to do that though because you basically have to be alert all night long.

PLEASE, PLEASE, PLEASE keep praying. This is getting sooooo hard (and I thought it was hard before!). Love you all.

Chapter Fourteen:
Hospice

• Friday, October 8, 2010 1:37 PM, EDT

They are in the process of admitting Tim to the Hospice unit. It will take a couple of hours, the doctors will know more this weekend but the feeling is less than two weeks. Tim is painfully trying to come to grips with this, pray and do whatever you need to and thanks.

What a day. It started off this morning with the doorbell ringing. It was Tim's former wife. She was apologetic as she had asked her son to let me know she was coming but he had forgotten to. Anyhow, she and Tim spent some time in the living room together. I have no idea what they talked about, but I am sure it was very healing for both of them. She was crying when she left. I felt sympathy for her but was so glad she had come over.

Later, Beth (Hospice nurse) came to check in on Tim. This was the grueling part. Tim was pacing the floor while he was talking to her. (The Colvins are known pacers.) He was asking her various questions like "Why is my stomach distended?" She would say "Because your body is filling up with fluid." Then he would say "Ok, what do we do about that?" And she would say "There is nothing we can do about that." And there were several questions just like that. I sat on the couch and watched him pace as he processed the answers to his questions. Then he stopped pacing. He looked her square in the face. He said "Oh my God, this is it. I really am dying, aren't I?" And she said "Yes, Tim, you are." I can barely even write about this. There are no words to describe what it is like to witness a human being coming to a realization such as this.

Then he said something that thoroughly surprised me. "Damn that Dr. Marco." I didn't even remember the name. When I questioned Tim, he reminded me that he was the first surgeon at Roswell that we met with who we thought would operate. He was the one that explained to us how dismal our situation was. "He said I had five to seven months and that son of a bitch was right." I hadn't even remembered any of that but when I later looked back at my notes, he was entirely accurate. Tim had not displayed much anger in the last five months, very little bitterness, and hardly any self-pity. This was one of the only statements like this he made. And I understood completely it was not the doctor truly, but the most classic case ever of "shoot the messenger."

Tim then turned to me and asked me in an accusing tone why I was so okay with this information. Wasn't I upset about it? This occurred one or two other times. I could immediately break down sobbing though and then he knew that I was just mustering up courage every moment of every day to cope with the knowledge that I was losing my husband. It was all a big front and he knew it.

Beth suggested that Tim go to the Hospice in-patient unit so that we could attempt to get him back on a regular sleep cycle. The lack of sleep was adding significantly to Tim's disorientation. Quite frankly, I felt it myself as well. I got more sleep than Tim, but not much more. I felt like I was on some loopy drugs at times. Tim did not want to go in-patient. He wanted to be home. I didn't blame him. He sat on the couch and I was in front of him, on my knees, looking into his eyes. I told him how much I loved him, but that I was unable to continue to take care of him on my own. I was exhausted beyond belief. But worse than that, he had fallen on my "shift" and I couldn't prevent him from hurting himself. I knew much worse could happen if he got a hold of his medicines. I realized from the physical position I was in, that I was on my knees, begging him to go to the hospital. And more importantly than that, I was begging him to forgive me for failing him in his 11th hour. Without all those words being said, we both knew what was meant. And he tenderly told me he would go, and I knew he forgave me for being human when I wanted to be so much more for him.

I now went into work mode. I knew I had to call all my clients and tell them I was taking a leave of absence. I had arranged with my supervisor to give them her number if they felt they needed sessions while I was out of commission. It was close to 30 calls for me to make. It never even occurred to me because of confidentiality that I could ask someone to make those calls for me. Plus by the time I gave up all those phone numbers, I could make the calls myself. So I started in. But I could hear Tim pacing again in the living room and his agitation was growing. At one point I heard him say angrily "What I need is MY WIFE. And I need her OFF THE PHONE." I would rush in and try to soothe him. I was trying to explain to him that I had to be away because once I got done with this, I would not ever have to leave him again. I would be DONE with work. So longer term gain for this short term pain of being without me. Looking back, hind sight is always 20/20. I wish so badly that I could take it back. I would have not left his side as he was trying to accept what was happening to him. I made the best decision I could in the moment with tremendous stress around me at all sides, but never the less, I am haunted by Tim's voice and my not being there for him.

At one point, Tim summoned Colin downstairs. He hooked arms with him and paced around the living room. I only caught snippets of their conversation. Tim told Colin "I am leaving now Colin." Colin said "Yeah, I know." And Tim said "No, I mean I am really leaving, for forever." And Colin said "Yeah, I know Dad." I'm not sure how many times that conversation was repeated, but it was a very poignant moment, and a very private one I felt odd about overhearing.

I had immediately called my family when the decision was made to take Tim in, and in normal form, they dropped everything and came to the house. My sister arrived before the ambulance came. Somehow, I had the presence of mind to ask Tim if he wanted to glance around the property he had worked so hard on over the last decade and he seemed delighted at the idea. Janet helped me dress him and get him ready. We put him in the wheelchair and pushed him around the different parts of the yard. We chatted a little bit about what it looked like when we bought it and all the changes and improvements we had made. While very emotional, I think Tim appreciated it.

When the ambulance came, I was very disappointed they would not let me drive with him. I thought about making a stink but decided to cooperate as Tim seemed able to handle it without me. What a day.

• Friday, October 8, 2010 10:36 AM
Guestbook entry from my high school friend
Darcy, Your journal entries just break my heart. I really wish I could absorb some of your pain. I'm thinking of you often, for whatever good that does. I hope you can get some rest and that there is a respite for Tim soon also.

• Friday, October 8, 2010 1:11 PM
Guestbook entry from our church family
Dear Tim and Darcy, You are remarkable people and your love for each other and for the world has touched many lives. Let God's love surround you during this time and always. We love you and are praying for you.

• Friday, October 8, 2010 1:21 PM
Guestbook entry from our church family
Darcy, Tim, and Frankie and family, I love you all and pray for you and please call us if you need help at a moment's notice.

• Friday, October 8, 2010 2:29 PM
Guestbook entry from Frankie's friend's family
Oh Darcy, I am so sorry. Hospice will be able to make Tim very comfortable. I pray for comfort and peace for Tim during this time. God bless you all so very much!

• Friday, October 8, 2010 3:36 PM
Guestbook entry from my high school friend
Our hearts ache for you. We're praying God gives you peace and strength. Much love and hugs.

• Friday, October 8, 2010 3:43 PM
Guestbook entry from my Chicago friend
Darcy, Tim and Frankie, You continue to be in our Mishaberach. A prayer for the healing of body, soul, heart and peace with all that lies ahead. I love your strength Darcy, but then I always have.

• Friday, October 8, 2010 5:10 PM
Guestbook entry from our church family
Oh Honey, my heart goes out to you, Tim and Frankie. You are constantly in my thoughts, Darcy. I so recall the day I took my mom to the Hospice unit. It was one of the hardest things I've ever done, but absolutely the right thing to do. It is also the safest for all of you, especially after what you've been through these past few days.

• Friday, October 8, 2010 7:16 PM
Guestbook entry from Frankie's friend's family
Darcy, I wish I could take some of your pain away. You and Tim are so brave and it is just heart wrenching hearing about this awful journey. Words cannot express how sorry I am that this is happening to Tim and your whole family.

• Friday, October 8, 2010 7:43 PM
Guestbook entry from Tim's cousin
Dear Tim and clan, I am very sorry to hear about your predicament. Know that you will be truly missed and heaven will be even better for your presence there. Selfishly however, we want you to remain here and make our lives brighter. I sincerely hope that your pain is tolerable and that you find some peace. Keep in mind that although we may not understand God's plan for our lives, He does indeed have a plan and if we trust in Him all will eventually be made clear to us. Anyway, know that you are deeply loved and thank you for sharing your life with us.

• Saturday, October 9, 2010 2:48 PM
Guestbook entry from our cyber friend
Darcy, Tim and family, Sending prayers for healing, comfort and understanding. The Lord knows what you need so I'll let Him figure out where to help, I'll just put in my order. Amen.

• Monday, October 11, 2010 7:38 AM, EDT

So very hard for me to even remember the course of events to update you all. Hospice has computers but none of them link to the internet. Everything has become such a blur but I will do my best to get information to you.

This continues to be a baffling roller coaster ride, only the ups and downs are more extreme and come more quickly. Bottom line, after reading labs, etc., Tim is suffering from delirium due to severe sleep deprivation. (I was getting close to that myself.) This is the most common reason people end up getting admitted (not pain or breathing issues but delirium) and also the toughest set of symptoms to treat and get under control. His sleep deprivation is caused somewhat by the disease, but more so by Tim's personality. His father died at a young age of cancer and he spent the end pacing the floor saying "I'll sleep when I'm dead." Tim outright has told us that he plans to repeat that pattern.

We (medical personnel, etc.) continue to try and explain to Tim that this attitude is detrimental to his health and will hasten his death. His body (like ours) must have an extended, solid sleep pattern at night. As of now, this is slowly improving with tweaked medication at night but it takes a while to get the right doses down. Plus because he was in this condition an entire week, it will take longer to correct. Doctor says that if he continues to do this wakefulness continuously, they will eventually have to heavily sedate him, which means he would no longer have responsive contact with others.

In addition, they discovered his hemoglobin is a third of what it should be which means his body is deprived of the oxygen it needs. (It is not the type of condition that can be resolved by just giving him oxygen, but he does have access to it whenever he feels he needs it.) There is no way to be sure how this condition developed but the best assumption is disease progression. The only resolution to this is a blood transfusion. If he got one, he would breathe a bit easier if it is successful. This would require a trip to the hospital by ambulance, then a return trip to Hospice. It basically takes all day.

At one point, Tim was coherent enough to have a conversation with the doctor and me about this. Of course there is no "right" medical decision regarding this so it came down to our preference. If Tim was able to make the decision himself, I am much more comfortable with that. Tim said his priority is coherency. The only thing that will help that is sleep control. So we are going to fix that first, then he will face the decision about the transfusion. So we are looking for solid sleep most of the night; then it has to stay that way. After discussing his night last night, we will revisit this conversation.

I have to get back to the Hospice unit. These are the facts, how Tim has been living this out is another very long entry but also very important to this whole story. So next time I get to a computer I will attempt to write that aspect of it. Don't even have time to check typos so do me a favor and overlook them ☺.

By the way, Tim is in room 131. Visiting hours are 24/7.

127

Once again, there were a few people who offered to stay at Hospice to give me a break. It was such a dilemma for me. Things were changing by the minute so I hated to miss any second with him. I already had to be gone on Saturday, the morning after he had been admitted. For whatever reason, I had decided it would be a good idea to highlight my hair. Unfortunately, I streaked it orange-red and needed it fixed in a desperate way. I had someone to do it, but it took a couple of hours. Tim had people call me every half hour or so. He was so upset that I wasn't there. My nerves were completely shot by the time I returned. I truly wanted to not leave his side, but I have a son to take care of also. And I'm supposed to take care of myself somehow so I can continue to care for everyone else. It was maddening.

Some of Tim's family came in for a shift. It was quite stressful. They hadn't been there for awhile and when they walked in, it felt like they were thinking we had no idea how to care for Tim. My family that had been keeping close vigil was devastated by their comments. They (Tim's family) thought the room was dirty and demanded housekeeping be brought in (at 9:00 PM). They were upset that Tim was lying there uncovered and exposed. (That's ok, they would soon discover that Tim would remove anything on him within minutes if they tried to dress him again.) I was somewhat used to their demeanor, but when I tried to explain what things were agitating to Tim, I was told "WE can handle his moods" and cut off from further conversation.

That upset me. It really had nothing to do with what I could handle, or anyone else. It had to do with the medical plan we had set up carefully with his doctor. Tim's agitation was keeping him from resting. And his lack of rest was going to hasten his death. I wasn't trying to keep him from being angry because I couldn't handle his moods. I drove home bawling. However, I actually had a conversation on the phone with the Hospice staff. They were wonderful as always. They saw everything going on and knew how dedicated my family and I were. They actually asked me if I wanted to have them removed from Tim's care. I said no, that in spite of their manner, they loved Tim and wanted to be part of his care. Hospice made it crystal clear that I was Tim's wife and that at any time if I became uncomfortable, they would step in and intervene. They made me feel so much better. I guess because an "objective" entity validated me and my family. It was obvious to them how much we cared for Tim and advocated for his life at every moment. They understood the big picture.

The irony didn't escape me. Some of Tim's family resented me and felt like I wasn't good for him. Maybe they even felt I tried to keep them from him. The actual truth was, I was the one that insisted Tim's family have their time with him. In spite of how they disliked me, I guarded their relationship with Tim. I might have gone home and cried my eyes out, but I didn't stop them from being with him.

• **Monday, October 11, 2010 3:52 PM**
Guestbook entry from Frankie's teacher

Thanks for the update! I keep thinking of Frankie and praying for him, and am drawn to Jeremiah 29:11: "For I know the thoughts that I think toward you, saith the Lord, thoughts of peace, and not of evil, to give you an expected end." I believe that Jesus will be holding him through all of this, and please know that I will do whatever I can. Frankie has been blessed with so many gifts and such a loving family! I am praying that Tim can get a good night's rest, and maybe you can too! God bless.

• **Monday, October 11, 2010 9:46 PM**
Guestbook entry from Tim's family's friend

My prayers continue to be with all of you... but especially you, Darcy. I know exactly how difficult this is... let others do for you so you can spend as much time as possible with Tim. Surround yourself with those that love you both... and try to let God do the rest.

• **Tuesday, October 12, 2010 6:42 AM, EDT**

Computers are still down at Hospice. I just snuck home for a couple of hours to try and get some things caught up...

There is no way to even explain how the days go. Tim has been "the man with a plan," or the guy with surprises. Unless you have spent some time at Hospice, I probably can't give you a clear picture. Tim goes in extremes — like near death, then suddenly sits up and wants a meal to eat. There have been some very, very funny moments. Like our minister coming to give us both communion. We were gathered in a large semi-circle and the sniffles filled the room. After the wine, Tim looked up and said "I'd like a chaser." The room went from sacred and somber to everyone cracking up...

Or the time he told me he wants to be buried in a hat — NOTHING else. Eventually he let me know what he wanted to wear but we got a good chuckle out of that.

As far as I go, Tim can go from needing me directly in front of him at all times, to telling the family to "Please announce her before she comes in the room, she tries to micro-manage me..."

It is exhausting — on every level possible. Tim has a few times now verbalized a clear plan for accepting his death, not hanging on, and asking why he can't go home to be with God. There are times the doctor was convinced he was on his way and then he would shoot up in bed again.

Yesterday he was able to verbalize he wishes to be in a sleep state. The doctor feels he has spoken this in many ways but his body just isn't cooperating. She is hoping to help his body catch up to his wishes.

Monday morning brought an entirely different day. He barely woke all day, when he did he insisted on getting up to go to the bathroom. He is like dead weight now, no more following behind him as he slowly shuffles. He is too weak to even stand. For the first time, I can't understand what his groans mean. This part has been very hard for me to accept. Yesterday I found out his job has taken his voice mail off and assigned his phone to someone else. Of course this was the right thing to do but it nearly broke my heart. I guess I wanted to be able to call it and still hear his dedicated voice.

So we will see what tomorrow brings. You are still welcome to come any time, day or night, but the atmosphere has changed from somewhat jovial to keeping a very, very quiet environment for him.

I am trying to attach information. Let me know if I am successful. We have been selected as a benefit recipient on the 16th (how wonderful and humbling for us!) and they'd like us to invite everyone on their behalf. Not sure if I will be able to make an appearance or not...

Also, if anyone wants to borrow Taffy... she is quite lonely and out of sorts... love you all.

I don't have a ton of regrets about this time period with Tim, but there is one that occurred this week at Hospice. I was on top of most things regarding him. I always asked questions, knew the medical plan, and knew what medicines he was getting and why. One night when I was by myself with Tim, two nurses came in that I hadn't seen before, which meant they hadn't taken care of Tim before either. They came in with two shots for him. I asked what they were. I explained to them that he had that medicine before but it was given to him through his mediport. They informed me that I was misinformed. That medicine was not even available in that form. I argued with them, quite certain of what I was saying. I got the old "I have been working here 20 years and that medicine has never been available in mediport form." They were so adamant and condescending, I actually caved and assumed I was wrong. I watched helplessly as they had to move Tim on his side to give him the shot. Tim moaned in pain as I cringed. Then to my horror they had to move him completely to the other side for the second shot. More pain for him. I was in tears. I couldn't wait until they were done and I could climb back in bed with him and comfort him.

As they left, I again asked them to re-check their records. A couple of hours later, the nurse returned and said that she was surprised to find out that I was indeed correct. I was so disgusted with them. How dare they walk in on a shift and adopt such a-know-it-all attitude? How dare they walk into a shift and not carefully read their patient's records? But that was nothing compared to the disgust I felt with myself. I am Tim's advocate. I knew in my heart what I thought was right, but I let them intimidate me. And Tim suffered because I wimped out.

Now I know in the scheme of things, this was a relatively small thing. But it was monumental in my mind. I resolved again to never doubt my instincts and fight even harder next time. I knew I was wearing out but this was no time for slacking in fortitude.

• Tuesday, October 12, 2010 8:11 AM
Guestbook entry from Tim's former colleague
Tim, People have kept our office updated on your journey. They are good friends! We made it to your benefit, but you had already left. There was a corner of employees, laughing and remembering all the good times we had. Wish you were there for that part, the connections we have made will last a lifetime, and you are part of those precious memories. Still hard to grasp your illness. I will always remember you from when I first started 23 years ago, so young, full of life and quick witted. (I think we all view ourselves as if we were still 25.)

Still marvel at the wallpaper job you did in our foyer. You said the transition piece that wrapped up the stairwell was the most difficult piece you had ever done. You did it perfectly, and I always point it out to guests. Well, my friend, I hope it goes well and I will see you again!

• Tuesday, October 12, 2010 9:39 AM
Guestbook entry from my high school friend's parents
Darcy and Tim, As you know, the journey can be mystifying, frightening, ever-changing, and most emotional... find time to step back for a moment... take a 15 minute time out... treat yourself to a specialty coffee/tea and a forbidden pastry/donut/dessert... close your eyes... and thank God for being there along the way.

• Wednesday, October 13, 2010 7:34 AM, EDT

Home again briefly to try and catch up on the absolute necessities...

Frankie is hanging in there. He is finally starting to talk more to me. He has been scared and worried and we have been trying to talk through it...

Tim has not woken up in a significant way since Monday morning. He does wake up to go to the bathroom every few hours. Incontinence has started but he seems to be aware of this after it happens. The bathroom issues are paramount to him so it has been quite a struggle. He is not strong enough to stand, and barely can sit up but somehow he communicates that he insists on getting up for the bathroom. I think he even has the staff baffled.

Yesterday at supper time he had not awakened for several hours, then he woke up, yelled at me, and pushed me. (Why? Because I wasn't getting him to the bathroom fast enough.) What a stinker! Of course, I realize he isn't doing any of it on purpose but the whole thing is just so damned hard to keep living through.

His daughter Emily is coming Thursday from Georgia. Some of you have asked how to pray. I truly believe it is ok to start praying that God will take him. He has breathed out short sentences like "Why can't I go home to God" and others that indicate he is truly ready but his body won't cooperate. This is a situation where his young age is working against him. So if you are comfortable, please pray that he will achieve the peace needed to pass on to the next life; one where there will be no imperfect bodies; one where he will see the parents (including my mom) that he misses so dearly...

Love you all.

• **Wednesday, October 13, 2010 11:55 AM, EDT**

Hello from the Hospice unit. Yeaaaah! The internet is up...

I spoke with the doctor this morning (she's wonderful by the way). She said there is once again a definite change in Tim. He will not be responsive anymore, most likely though, he can still hear. He moans on occasion which is usually to let us know he is wet. We are continuously giving him reassuring messages that we all are here, love him, and that his family will be taken care of.

He is only on the methadone and the steroid at this point. He needs no sleep aids. They are relatively certain the moaning is not from pain as he has not been in pain for almost the entire process.

The doctor said I didn't need to make that frantic phone call, but this is clearly end stages. Emily is doing her best to get here today, worst case she will be here tomorrow...

If anyone has a CD with mellow piano music, I think he would enjoy that. The nurses say that often relaxes them. When we went to Niagara on the Lake he thoroughly enjoyed a piano CD in the room. So don't hesitate at this point if you want to come. Soon another transition will occur where he probably will not want to be touched or hovered over anymore. That will so break my heart when I sense he doesn't want me to lie next to him anymore.

• Wednesday, October 13, 2010 8:41 PM, EDT

I came home briefly to spend some awake time with Frankie...

When I left, they had given Tim some sleeping medicines. He had been groaning some and starting to look a little uncomfortable (although not in pain). Once he was settled, they put a catheter in. He asked for it to be removed on Saturday but I thought it was time to give it another shot. He is so stressed by his need to go to the bathroom. I am hoping this will relieve more of his anxiety.

I have been meeting some with our church staff regarding upcoming arrangements. If anyone has any interest at all in doing a reading, saying a prayer, or reading a favorite story for the service, please let me know in the next couple of days. I am not requesting anyone do so, but don't want to shut anyone out who has something on their heart and wants to contribute in this way...

Love you all...

• Wednesday, October 13, 2010 7:52 AM
Guestbook entry from our church family

Good Morning, Darcy, You are truly inspirational. All of us are indeed praying for Tim, but also for you. Truly, throughout the day, my conversations with God reflect just what you expressed in your message this morning.

• Wednesday, October 13, 2010 8:02 AM
Guestbook entry from Mom B

Tim, You have my prayers for a wonderful journey 'home'. Love, Mom B.

• Wednesday, October 13, 2010 10:07 AM
Guestbook entry from my high school friend

Hi Darcy. I have quietly kept up on your journal and Tim's progress but today felt like I just needed to reach out to you.

I pray comfort for you in a time that I cannot even imagine. I know that your faith in God will help you through this, but at the same time please remember how many people (friends and family) love you guys and are keeping you close in our hearts. I pray for Tim's last days to be as peaceful and pain-free as possible and that you can also find comfort in that.

• Wednesday, October 13, 2010 11:24 AM
Guestbook entry from our church family

Dear Darcy, I am praying for both of you. Be strong. God loves you and is so proud of both of you.

• Wednesday, October 13, 2010 11:41 AM
Guestbook entry from my clients

Dear Darcy, Tim, and family, We continue to pray that God will give you ALL an increased awareness of His presence with you. He is always with us, but at times we are blessed with a greater awareness of His presence. That has been and continues to be our prayer for all of you as God continues to reveal His plans. Jeremiah 29:11 is a promise and statement of fact!

Interesting choice of verse to offer, the same one Frankie's teacher sent. I know the people who sent it this time are also people of great faith. And people of great faith even after living through heartbreaking adversity, over and over again. I have no idea what words like "hope" and "future" even mean anymore, but I have faith that we will figure it out and that God will walk beside us as we do.

• Wednesday, October 13, 2010 12:03 PM
Guestbook entry from my supervisor
Hi Darcy, I'm wordless but here for you in any way you can think of...

• Wednesday, October 13, 2010 1:10 PM
Guestbook entry from my college friends
HI Darcy, I read your posts every time you send them. So does my husband. I wish we could be there with you in body as well as spirit. I am glad you have a local support system to stand by you, watch your cat, bring CD's, do benefits, etc. God bless you and Tim, Frankie and the rest of the family. We love you and will continue to pray you feel God's closeness to you.

• Wednesday, October 13, 2010 3:23 PM
Guestbook entry from Frankie's friend's family
Darcy, Thinking of you every second and praying often that God sends his angels to guide Tim home. Those are the prayers you want so I will do my best to keep them coming. Continue to talk to Tim and hold him near for as long as he will let you. Please take care.

• Wednesday, October 13, 2010 9:43 PM
Guestbook entry from our church family
Dear Darcy, I don't know what else to say tonight, other than the fact that you are loved by many, many family members and dear friends who wish they could do something meaningful for you at this time. Whatever you need, of course you know, you can ask me.

Chapter Fifteen

He is gone...

Chapter Sixteen:
Rituals

• Thursday, October 14, 2010 11:27 PM, EDT

Funeral Home Visiting Hours: Saturday, 2:00 PM - 4:00 PM
and 7:00 PM - 9:00 PM; Georgian Funeral Home

Funeral Service at our church; Sunday 2:00 PM.

Sorry for such briefness; I will do better when I can somehow
breathe again...

Not only did Tim choose his cemetery plot and design his head stone, he also selected his funeral home. He picked out the casket, lining, and everything else that goes with it. I thought at one point he had written his obituary. Unfortunately, when the time came, the funeral home was booked like mad. We would have had to wait several days to use the funeral home we had chosen. That wouldn't have been so bad in and of itself, but if we did that, Emily and her family could not have attended. So I found myself having to do things quickly and somewhat in a panic. We went to our second choice for funeral homes and luckily they were available. However, the first person had never typed up all of our preferences so I had to try and select everything all over again. I found myself being ridiculously crabby about this. I did not want to spend my time and energy doing this, especially just five hours after Tim taking his last breath. And I could not find his obituary for the life of me so I had to rewrite it. It was ok, but I did not think to mention his employment which was really disappointing considering how much Tim loved his job. It was the funeral home's job to ask the right questions, but they had fallen short on many key points. In the big scheme of things, none of it matters I guess. Probably felt better to direct my anger and upset somewhere else besides dealing with the fact that I had lost my partner.

• Thursday, October 14, 2010 1:18 PM
Guestbook entry from my supervisor
I'm so sorry Darcy. I hope as you grieve the loss of him and his love for you that you can also celebrate his life...

- **Thursday, October 14, 2010 1:25 PM**
Guestbook entry from Frankie's friend's family
Darcy and family, We are so saddened by this. You are in our thoughts and prayers. Love you.

- **Thursday, October 14, 2010 1:49 PM**
Guestbook entry from my friend
My dear Darcy, He is at peace and in a warm, loving and better place. My heart is crying with you, but also glad Tim suffers no more. You've been through so much, and more lies ahead. Hold fast to those who love you and surround you. Faith, family and friends will guide you through.

- **Thursday, October 14, 2010 1:54 PM**
Guestbook entry from my high school friend
My heart aches for you, my dear friend. How blessed you are to have had each other and Frankie. Tim leaves behind a truly wonderful legacy in his family. Still praying for all of you. I love you, Darc.

- **Thursday, October 14, 2010 2:31 PM**
Guestbook entry from Frankie's friend's family
Darcy, I am so saddened by Tim's passing. I know that he has finally made his journey home to God and is now in a place where he will be reunited with all the people he has lost throughout his life and will no longer be plagued with any sickness. Tim wanted so badly to stay with you and the children for many years. Cherish the memories you have made with him over the years and may you and your family find peace and comfort.

- **Thursday, October 14, 2010 3:05 PM**
Guestbook entry from Tim's colleague
So sorry to hear of Tim's passing today. He was a terrific person and will be greatly missed. It's so unfortunate that someone who so loves life, family, friends, work, sports, etc. goes at such a young age. I will take comfort in knowing that I will see him and laugh with him again someday. My heart goes out to Tim's family in this time of sadness. In loving prayer.

• Thursday, October 14, 2010 6:57 PM
Guestbook entry from my high school friends
Dearest Darcy and family, My heart goes out to all of you at this most difficult time. Tim and you are all truly loved. Even though taken far too young, he obviously has lived a full life of happiness and knew what matters most in life. Please know that we are holding you close in our hearts and prayers. May this and the support of all others in your life provide you some comfort. Much love and the deepest of sympathy.

• Thursday, October 14, 2010 9:10 PM
Guestbook entry from Tim's cousin
Tim is my beloved cousin whom I will miss dearly. I love you, Tim and my favorite picture will always be the picture of you, me, and our cousin at our last 2010 family reunion. What a blessing to have that beautiful picture. I love and I miss you. I will see you when God calls me home. My faith and love of our heavenly God promised that your pain, fear, and suffering have all gone away. This is the joy and hope I cling to for you as I did for my mom. Darcy, I love you and my prayers continue for you and your little one. Children know little of pain and suffering when they are young and well loved. You are a wonderful mom. Please remember that it is now that God is carrying you and cradling you in His arms. You are the apple of God's eyes. To all Tim's children I love you and you would be my second cousins and we may not know each other very well. I loved your dad dearly and he talked of how proud he was of all of you.

• Thursday, October 14, 2010 10:49 PM
Guestbook entry from Tim's niece
When you passed away I cried but I am glad you are in a better place and in no more pain. I love you Uncle Tim! You will be missed.

• Friday, October 15, 2010 7:26 AM, EDT

I just wanted to let you know a little bit about Tim's last day...

He was pretty quiet throughout the day. His small arm or leg gestures seemed to stop. (He would sometimes pull off his sheet or want the "brief" off that he was wearing.)

140

He would sometimes moan, although they still were confident this was not due to pain. His breathing was steady. He did however let out these very long, loud sighs. (They would totally startle me if I was lying next to him.) Our minister was there and later told me he was reminded of the verses in Romans where it talks about the Spirit groaning on our behalf...

About 12:30 PM (I really have little concept of time) we decided to freshen him up. He was breathing rhythmically but seemed to be moaning. I always check with a nurse or doctor to make sure he doesn't need something for a better restful state. They gave him some sleep medicine and sent the doctor in. She reassured us she had checked his lungs and they were perfectly clear. She said the sounds were carbon dioxide release and nothing to be concerned about...

After she left the room most people dispersed to get lunch, etc. I leaned over into Tim's ear and told him "Holy cow Tim, that doctor was a hottie. You would have liked her!" (She was very beautiful.)

Probably not five minutes later I was in the room with just a couple of people (not even sure exactly who they all were) and I noticed Tim's eyes were open. I looked and said "I don't think he's breathing." (After you have a microscopic eye on someone for five months you notice every little thing.) Those in the room said of course he was breathing. Tim's cousin said to put my hand on his heart and feel it beating... I told her I didn't feel anything.

I ran down the hall to the nurses' station. On the way, I yelled into the waiting room that I thought Tim was gone, everyone jumped up in shock...

The nurse came right down and confirmed with surprise that he indeed was gone.

My legs buckled underneath me. When you've been on a journey like this, it seems ridiculous to say we were all shocked. But we were! He didn't do anything by the book — he never did and especially not during this illness. They called him the surprise guy and he remained that right to the end.

I was standing at the side of the bed. There were several people waiting in silence, all with shocked looks on their faces. Dad was next to me. We were all holding our breath as the nurse attempted to find a heartbeat. She looked up at me and shook her head. My legs truly did buckle and I grasped for my father to hold me up. I can't even explain what went through my head in a matter of seconds. The biggest thing was "I really couldn't do it. I really couldn't keep him alive." But then at the same time I knew all that we had been transformed into and knew the goal wasn't to keep him alive at all. So many complicated thoughts flashed through me. All that came out of my mouth was "NO!!" as I moaned and desperately held onto Dad. And Dad did what dads do — tried to fix it and snap me out of it. I don't remember the exact words he said, but something along the lines of "Ok, get it together."

It actually infuriated me. Another torrent of words swept through my mind. "WHAT?? ARE YOU KIDDING ME? I have been a tower of strength for over five months. I have been strong for Tim and everyone else. WHEN DO I GET TO FALL APART??" Visions of women in black tearing their clothes and wailing out loud came into view. Can't I be like that? But alas, all that happened was I straightened myself up and wept quietly with everyone else.

I had it all figured out. I knew from my mom's death that especially with Hospice care, they tell you when to make that urgent call to everyone to come before it is too late. I knew his breathing would begin to slow and the room would be packed as we quietly and peacefully waited for that last breath.

Shows you what I know.

Emily arrived within minutes after her dad died. She was totally fine with that. She is convinced he waited until she had landed and felt like she was still there. Our grandson Parker knew exactly who Grampy was. He would take people by the hand and point to him and say "owie."

The principal brought Frankie to Hospice for us. Frankie said he was very glad that Parker came the day daddy died because it helped him not be sad.

So now I get to live with my last words to my husband being

about his hot doctor. Everyone who knows us thinks it was a perfect last exchange... gotta have that sense of humor. We've all agreed — it just doesn't seem real, not at all. And I know that is normal. And then it is so real that my knees buckle all over again.

It was so strange to walk out of the building. It felt like we had been there for months, and these people who walk this incredibly difficult journey with you are suddenly gone, never to be seen again. And those not on that particular shift you don't get to say bye to at all. It is all so bizarre.

As much as Tim and I planned in advance, today will still be a terribly busy day. Know when you see him, attend the service, or whatever, that even if things seem a little out of the ordinary, Tim picked most things out himself... Of course, I tend to think a little outside of the box myself... is that an understatement?

• Friday, October 15, 2010 7:36 AM
Guestbook entry from our church family
Dear Darcy, Over the next several days and weeks, you will feel great love and caring from so many people who want to be there for you and Frankie. Although of course, I didn't know Tim nearly as well as your close friends and family, I felt a change in him, even toward someone like me. The last three or four times I saw Tim, he'd come up and HUG me with a big smile. That is the Tim I will remember, especially knowing that he was a shy man. So, telling him his doctor is a hottie as your last words: PRICELESS. See you soon.

• Friday, October 15, 2010 8:45 AM
Guestbook entry from my friend
Knowing Tim as I did, I think the last exchange was very much him ☺. I also believe that his passing the way he did was "his way," a way to surprise and do things differently. You're right. He was determined to do that to the end. Although a surprise, it sounds like his last moments were peaceful and I'm glad for that. In my eyes, he won his "battle" and is now at home.

• Friday, October 15, 2010 11:28 AM
Guestbook entry from Frankie's friend's family
Darcy, Thank you so much for sharing Tim's last day with us. You know, you think a lot like me... I probably would fill my husband in on the hot doctor as well. So you are not totally out of the norm... or maybe I am out of the box right with you. I miss you tons in my life and my family enjoyed the times that we were able to share with you and Tim. Maybe when things settle down some, I hope you and I could get together. Tim told me to do that at his fundraiser at Friendly's. Actually, he whispered it in my ear right after he said my family should come over swimming and no suits were needed. That is the last laugh that Tim Colvin had given me. My response back to him was I only wanted him to have happy memories and our family skinny dipping in his pool would be a scary one. He laughed and it made me feel really good. I do hope this story gives you a little chuckle during such a very sad time.

• Friday, October 15, 2010 12:25 PM
Guestbook entry from Tim's friend
That was beautiful to read!

• Friday, October 15, 2010 4:33 PM
Guestbook entry from our cyber friend
Darcy, My prayers go out to you, Frankie, Emily and the rest of the family. There aren't enough words to take away the lost feelings, but know that Tim isn't in any pain any longer. Sending angels to hug and hold you all.

• Friday, October 15, 2010 9:02 PM
Guestbook entry from our church family
Darcy, My wife and I convey our deepest sympathies to you in your loss. As difficult as it has been, we know that the Lord was in charge throughout the process. We admire your courage and faith during this incredibly difficult time for you and your family. We have followed from afar and you and Tim have been in our daily prayers. I know that you will have the prayers and loving support of a great community of people, all tied together in their love for our Lord.

144

Of course I didn't know it at the time I read Jill's entry, but just about
two weeks later, her husband would pass away in the Hospice room
across the hall from where Tim's was. Her husband battled cancer
longer than we did, and I don't think they had even a small fraction
of the support that we did. What a brave woman. YOU are a great
teacher also, my friend.

• Saturday, October 16, 2010 8:28 AM, EDT

Do you all remember awhile ago when we worked so hard
to get the name of the patient that had the same diagnosis?
Rose and her husband Wyatt invited us into their home and
shared their journey with us.

About a month ago, she called us and spoke with Tim about
how he made the decision to continue treatment or switch to
palliative care. It was so nice to hear from her.

Yesterday, Wyatt called; Rose passed away on Tuesday! He
had seen our notice in the paper. I was so pleased he called
but so terribly saddened. I still have goosebumps just thinking
about it. What are the chances they would both pass within two
days of each other? We promised to get together for tea in the
near future to discuss our journeys and the paths that lie ahead.

Those of you who believe in serendipity, divine appointments,
or whatever, will appreciate that story.

It was now time for the funeral home. I've had plenty of experience
with this over the years. There were a couple of ironies about this
day that hit me. The calling hours are on October 16th. That was the
original date the benefit was scheduled. We had decided to move
it up in case Tim wasn't feeling well by October. Never, ever in my
wildest dreams would I have thought that Tim would be gone by then.
That never crossed my mind. Now, instead of a party, we are hosting
funeral home hours.

October 16th is also Sweetest Day this year. In all honesty, Tim was
much better at the romantic stuff than I was. He sometimes said he had
the "girl memory" and I had the "boy memory." Like he kept a beverage
napkin from the bed and breakfast where we spent our wedding night.
Anyhow, somehow I recognized Saturday as Sweetest Day and then
I recognized that Sweetest Day, 2000 is the day that Tim proposed to
me. He had a tin box of chocolates (smart man) and a small stuffed
puppy dog that held the ring. A great memory. How bitter to be having
his funeral calling hours on the same day exactly one decade later.

When I told our daughter Emily, she slipped right into action. Tim had
intended on making his own picture boards for the funeral home. He
had started printing out shots he wanted, but our computer program
ran into a glitch I just couldn't get fixed in a timely fashion. Then Tim just
plain ran out of energy. All of Tim's older kids have their father's artistic
talent. Emily was especially good at collages so she locked herself up
into my office and went to work. She did a phenomenal job of course, but
she made a special Sweetest Day board of just Tim and I. It was lovely.

My sisters and friend took me shopping yesterday for something to
wear. I am glad we figured out what Tim was wearing. He wanted a
t-shirt, jeans, sneakers and his Sabres hat. The hat didn't look right
so we set it next to him. My dad panicked when we walked into the
funeral home. "Where's his suit?" I was glad I could tell him Tim picked
his own clothes out so I didn't get any disapproving lectures. I know

146

people say things like "Oh, he or she looks so good" and it seems like a ridiculous thing to say about someone in a casket, but Tim really did look great. His looks had changed so much over the months as his weight went up and down. He looked just like the Tim we all knew and loved. And having those clothes on him was just perfect.

While we were getting ready at the house, about 15 minutes before we needed to leave, I suddenly let out a huge squeal. I had totally forgotten some very important things. The word-find book and flashlight! I quickly told my family the story and they looked at me like "Are you serious?" I told them I was dead serious, no pun intended. So they quickly got in their cars and ran to the store to get a word-find book and flashlight. I went to the computer and typed out a quick note to place in the casket, explaining why those things were included. Tim was able to give everyone one last chuckle as they walked by his casket to pay their respects.

We did the usual 2:00 PM - 4:00 PM and 7:00 PM - 9:00 PM calling hours. I have no idea how many people actually came, but I know the lines went out the door for the entire time period. I know people didn't even come in because of the wait. For the evening hours I got smart and let someone bring me wine and keep my cup filled for me ☺.

Just a couple of snafus. During the first set of hours, I found myself standing next to Sheila (Tim's first wife) and her husband. We have been "friendly" for several years now. Her family came over to the house this summer and had a barbecue to spend some time with Tim. Sheila came to the house the day Tim went into Hospice. But I had to admit I felt very awkward greeting people in front of the casket and then introducing them to Tim's first wife. Sheila is also extremely shy and I'm quite sure she didn't relish being in that position either. I finally said something and Sheila and her husband left the line. Later I found out that I really upset my daughter (step-daughter for clarification purposes). She felt like her father had just died and she needed her mother by her side. I understood how she felt and was sorry she was upset, but I understood how I felt too. I just couldn't handle it along with everything else I was dealing with. Not at Tim's casket. Emily eventually forgave me, but it's one of those stories we will just never agree on.

As things were clearing out, I could sense there was some sort of conflict going on. For the most part, people tried to keep things away from me, figuring I had enough to deal with burying my husband. The problem is, when you are a therapist, you are pretty keen at picking up vibes — apparently even when you are exhausted. There were some flowers delivered to the funeral home from someone close to one of Tim's family members. (I didn't know the sender personally.) So those family members felt that the flowers belonged to them and wanted to take them home. When I figured out what was going on, I approached them and said they could take "their" flowers as well as any others that were there.

At some point in the night, I remembered that tonight was the other benefit being held where we were one of two recipients. I decided that I wanted to make an appearance. My sister and brother-in-law took me, and Tim's nephew and girlfriend came too. I was so grateful to them, especially Tim's family. It was really nice to have someone there to represent his side of the family. We didn't stay long but had a couple of drinks and chatted with some people I knew. The organization ended up paying our mortgage for a month or two. In spite of the day's activities, I had to tally some on the sweet side as well.

• **Sunday, October 17, 2010 5:38 PM**
Guestbook entry from Tim's cousin
Darcy and kids, God bless you all and may He hold you tenderly and safely in His hand as you begin another journey forward.

I know Tim will cherish you from above and be within you, as I feel those I have lost in my life even now. I vowed to celebrate those I have lost and see them in all the joys of life that I have before me, to celebrate their lives and cherish their memory. It has made healing more possible as time goes on. Please reach out to those who love you and desire to be there for you...Tim would want you to be comforted.

Something that has helped me with those passed on: "Although your ship sails from our sight, it does not mean the journey ends. It only means the river bends..." Much love.

Chapter Seventeen:
The Funeral Service

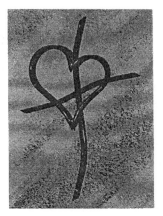

Timothy M. Colvin
October 17, 2010
2:00 p.m.

Sunday, October 17

The funeral service. There were many details to put together, but Tim and I had kept a list of the favorite verses and readings we had come across, knowing we could use them at his service. I didn't go to the regular worship service in the morning, but got dressed and ready to go to his afternoon funeral service in my new duds. I had a strange feeling, like I was getting ready for a date or something and actually felt kind of proud of how I looked. I arrived at the church and was ushered with my family to a waiting room to avoid the crowds. We were sitting around and chatting and I thought it bizarre how calm I actually was.

Then my body took over. The next thing I knew, I was in the exact position I was in five months earlier sitting in the surgeon's office. I knew I was passing out and was utterly out of control to do anything to stop it. It was the same odd thing, that I could hear the people around me talking but their voices were so, so distant. I couldn't speak. I knew they were getting cold cloths and I somehow had a vague sensation of the cool on my face. They were all trying to figure out where my anti-anxiety medicine was and if they could call someone to bring it to the church. In general, I have a better than average skill at knowing myself. This was one of the moments where I was completely and utterly clueless as to where I truly was. I thought I strangely had it together but my soul knew better. I literally just had to check out for a few moments.

Thankfully it passed relatively quickly so the service didn't have to be delayed much. It was an amazing service so I'm going to relate it to you piece by piece because it was beautiful and worth sharing.

To start with, Tim's former colleague and friend Chris sang a song and played guitar. Chris was in a band for a long time and Tim used to go often and hear him play. When the benefit came along, Chris got his band to play, which was of course very meaningful for us. They were delightful. He selected this piece as prelude music:

"May the rain fall soft upon your face until we meet again.
May God hold you in the palm of His hand."

After that, two of my girlfriends sang a song. Julie is in my band and women's quintet in our church. Tim thought she was adorable, like a Barbie doll he would say, with a sweet voice. Truth be told, Frankie had a crush on her for awhile too. Michelle was in the band at the church we were married in so we were old time friends and musicians together. The band sang in our wedding, and one of the pieces they performed was what I asked them to sing at Tim's funeral when we walked the casket down the aisle. We loved the words then and they were just as perfect at a funeral as they were at a wedding! It was written by Hans Peterson. I found out his father passed away in his 50's from cancer and was the inspiration for the lyrics.

"Everything is grace, as we see in others God's loving face.
Grateful people embrace even the pains in life, with God they turn and face.
Every moment we live by faith, every breath that we breathe is grace.
Everything that we live is grace.

Can we live with sorrow and with joy? With conflict and also peace?
Must a shade be only dark or light for us to keep our sanity?
Could it be that night and day and dancing and mourning are all a part of the same movement?

150

In the darkness there will be light. From its despair you will find hope. In your weakest moment there'll be strength. And out of death, new life is born. When you see the face of pain, find a home. Trust the promise you already know."

I had remembered the part about grace, but I had forgotten the verses and couldn't believe how perfect they were — the message of bitter and sweet that had become our mantra was in every verse of this song.

Our minister then welcomed everyone. "Good afternoon. My name is Reverend Miller and I am the pastor of this church, and along with my colleague Reverend Taylor and the staff of the church, I welcome you to this celebration of the life and witness of Tim Colvin. I know I speak for Darcy and on behalf of her family in thanking you for being here to celebrate Tim's life and for the hundreds of people that have gathered around them in the past months, have upheld them, and strengthened them on this journey that they have been on.

"What a fitting and appropriate song that every breath that we breathe is grace. I would ask us to take a moment and be aware of that grace in our own lives. Take a moment and draw in breath. Experience that as God's presence and know that surely God is here with us now. Let's take a moment of silence... Amen.

"For those of you that know Darcy, it shouldn't come as any surprise that this service is a reflection of not only Darcy, but Darcy and Tim, of people that have been special in their lives, of scriptures, and hymns, and words. So let us in this hour, let this service speak to us, and in some ways, speak for Tim as we gather to worship God."

Next, Tim's brother Roger did a reading, an invitation to worship. It came from the Roswell hospital prayer book. "In whatever state of mind you are, sing God's praises and set forth the greatness of the Creator. Whatever your feelings, reflect upon the Creator for everything. I offer myself in hymn of praise that brings peace everlasting. Day after day, He extends His care to everything He created. He will continue to do so forever. He who provides all. No one can measure the gifts of God. Who can appreciate the giver of them all?"

(As Tim and I devoured books together, we marked anything special we came across that we might want to use in the future for something like this. So when someone expressed an interest in speaking at the service, they were able to choose the one that most spoke to them.)

Our dear friend Sean read the Old Testament lesson. "A reading from Isaiah. Hast thou not known? Hast thou not heard, that the everlasting God, the Lord, the Creator of the ends of the earth, fainteth not, neither is weary? There is no searching of his understanding. He giveth power to the faint; and to them that have no might he increaseth strength. Even the youths shall faint and be weary, and the young men shall utterly fall. But they that wait upon the Lord shall renew their strength; they shall mount up with wings as eagles; they shall run, and not be weary; and they shall walk, and not faint."

The hymn that Tim chose surprised me, but when I heard it, I knew it was perfect. We had guitar rather than organ.

"Nearer my God to Thee, nearer to Thee.
Even though it be a cross, that raiseth me.
Still, all my song shall be — nearer my God to Thee, nearer to Thee.

Or if on joyful wing, cleaving the sky
Sun, moon and stars forgot, upward I fly
Still all my song shall be — nearer my God to Thee, nearer to Thee."

Next, one of Tim's childhood friends gave a brief reflection. He was someone I had never met until Tim got sick. When he heard the news, he and Tim re-connected. He brought over an Othello game they used to play regularly. It was amazing. They had written dates on the box when they played, and if I remember correctly, who won those games. He came over several times to see Tim with the goal of filling up that box. They were able to add several game dates to that box.

My sister Renee then did the New Testament reading. "A reading from the book of Romans. For as many as are led by the Spirit of God, they are the sons of God. For ye have not received the spirit of bondage again to fear; but ye have received the Spirit of adoption, whereby we cry, Abba, Father. The Spirit itself beareth witness with our spirit, that we are the children of God: And if children, then heirs; heirs of God, and joint-heirs with Christ; if so be that we suffer with him, that we may be also glorified together. For I reckon that the sufferings of this present time are not worthy to be compared with the glory which shall be revealed in us. For the earnest expectation of the creature waiteth for the manifestation of the sons of God. For the creature was made subject to vanity, not willingly, but by reason of him who hath subjected the same in hope, Because the creature itself also shall be delivered from the bondage of corruption into the glorious liberty of the children of God. For we know that the whole creation groaneth and travaileth in pain together until now. And not only they, but ourselves also, which have the firstfruits of the Spirit, even we ourselves groan within ourselves, waiting for the adoption, to wit, the redemption of our body."

(Yes, our bodies certainly need redeeming. No more cancer in heaven I presume.)

Chris sang another song at this point.
"Hear O Lord, the sound of my call. Hear O Lord and have mercy.
My soul is longing for the glory of You.
So hear O Lord, and answer me."

Our sister-in-law Sally then read another reading from Romans. "Likewise the Spirit also helpeth our infirmities: for we know not what we should pray for as we ought: but the Spirit itself maketh intercession for us with groanings which cannot be uttered. And He that searcheth the hearts knoweth what is the mind of the Spirit, because He maketh intercession for the saints according to the will of God. And we know that all things work together for good to them that love God, to them who are the called according to His purpose."

We selected this passage for so many reasons. Even though I am a graduate from Moody Bible Institute, I find that the older I get, the less sophisticated my prayers get. We did not know how to pray so many, many times. So it just became "Help us," several times a day, every day. And sometimes there weren't even those words. I would just cry and know God heard me. Secondly, in Tim's last hours, he would let these groans and sighs out that seemed to be out of the blue. They were long and not like anything I had ever heard from anyone before. They did not sound full of pain, but I couldn't quite describe what it touched in me. Lastly, I have heard that "All things work together for good" during most of my religious life. I had understood it to mean that God had a plan for our lives that we had to trust and accept, knowing it would all be "good" in the end. That theology has changed over the years for me. I now believe that with our free will, God kind of "co-creates" our lives with us as we make the choices we do. I don't think God "planned" for Tim to have cancer because it was for our own good. But I do understand that there is "good" in everything, even the darkest of things. There is sweet to savor in even the most bitter medicines.

Next, our Hospice chaplain spoke. We had requested she be on our care team because she attended our church and was a familiar face. She was so dear to our hearts as she watched our journey unfold. She spoke to us often about the transformation our marriage was experiencing, so I asked her to speak.

"My name is Nina and I'm a chaplain at Hospice and was called to be on the in-home care team that provided compassionate care to Tim, to Darcy, and to the family. In her poem entitled 'When Death Comes,' Mary Oliver concludes that when she dies, she wants to be able to say 'I have not just visited the earth.' As chaplain at Hospice, I witness patients and families pressed, and pressed down hard to consider whether they have merely been visitors to their life, whatever the length of their days. Or have they been pilgrims in life? Not all patients pursue this question. Few do it willingly. But when dying and death comes, as it does for all of us, some will dare to walk the stoney path, the twilight road, to plumb not just the meaning of their life, nor wonder about the future. Some choose to be fully awake in and to the present moment, the present breath, the present light, the present touch, the present hope.

"What I heard, and what I saw when visiting Tim and Darcy in their home, was courage to grab that taut, plumb line, placed before them by a cruel disease and a more cruel prognosis. They dared assess the boundaries and current limits of their marriage, shaped as it was by habit and accommodation of their life together. And then adjusting to new demands that terminal illness always brings. I witnessed them establishing and living into new patterns of communication, that were unimaginable a year ago. Recommitting their days, each moment if necessary, becoming awake to their individual lives and their life together. They discovered a depth of abundance which surprised them. And for those of us that had the honor of being close to them, surprised even us.

"Yes, hearts were breaking. I heard them shatter, more than once, knowing as they did, there would be no 60th wedding anniversary celebration. Yet I also heard something else — the breath of transformation, giving them life, birthing them, creating them into something new. I saw tears rain down their cheeks as they negotiated the painful path, the push-pull of life, together as Tim wrestled with how he would live his dying. How Darcy expressed her needs and hope in all this. I saw them touch and talk and cry and hold each other in such intimate ways, that I will forever be changed by it. And live into that hope of what is possible in marriage, in commitment to one another. Those of us gathered here today are not just mere people who believe in change, resolutions, rather we are people of transformation. We follow the One who has been, and is being now transformed into a new life, into a new community, that even death will not defeat. We are people of transformation. We believe it. We live it. We are it.

"Transformation is hard, hard, hard work. Change is easy, transformation takes our whole life. It takes our mind. It takes our heart. It takes our spirit. It even takes our body. That's what we come here today to remember and celebrate, that we are people of transformation. And I saw in my brief moments with Darcy and Tim and the family, a breath of transformation. A breath that this world needs so much, that marriages need and crave so much.

"So I am here to tell you, my dear friends, that Darcy and Tim did not merely visit their marriage. Rather, they sojourned in it with courage and humility and vulnerability. And something new has come. So I say to you, Darcy, and to my friend Tim — Well done! Well done, good and faithful servants, Amen."

Next my dear, dear friend Summer spoke. Words cannot describe how invaluable she was every step of the way, but especially in pulling everything together for the funeral and luncheon.

"Life has beginnings and endings and then there is that in-between time called 'living.' Some people fit a lot of living in a shorter space of time than others. From May 7th until October 14th, Tim Colvin lived a lot of his life and with a different purpose in mind than before. For the next 160 days, he began a journey of living strong. In Tim's first CaringBridge journal entry of June 9th, he professes to be an independent, do everything himself, Mr. Workaholic. And for those of you who knew him best; that apparently may have been an understatement! He wrote at that time that he fully intended to fight for his life, scratching, clawing and kicking. I would say that initially that seemed to be the case; however that kind of living takes more energy than is reasonably sustainable and so that is where the transformation of Tim began to take shape.

"The do-it-yourselfer guy became the one that other people did things for and that requires a humbling of spirit in order for that to happen gracefully. While Tim concentrated on learning how to live with cancer, the rest of the family learned how to shoulder responsibilities so Tim could concentrate on his health. Prior to Tim's diagnosis they decided to refurbish the pool and backyard. The decision to forge ahead with those plans became the first of many things that were placed on Tim's "Bucket List." He wanted to be able to enjoy the pool as he had in the past with his family but more importantly, for his family to be able to enjoy it when he was gone and remember all the happy times together. Finishing the yard became a labor of love that Tim could only watch as family, friends and church family completed it for him. In another CaringBridge journal entry Tim wrote, 'Just when I think that Darcy doesn't have any more in the tank to give, she seems to have an uncanny persistence of heart and mind to make the impossible into possible. I love you, honey.' Remember that this was not a personal love note to his wife for just her to read... he put that out there for everyone on CaringBridge to see. Not just a romantic gesture but a genuine and articulate appreciation for Darcy for all of us to witness.

"Normally a very private man, Tim's battle with cancer now became public, which also garnered a showing of support and hope for him and his family that sets a huge precedence. In case you don't already know this about Tim and Darcy, I'll let you in on the worst kept secret ever — they are both huge planners and organizers. From the basement to the yard, everything has a place and by golly it better be in it! Only those of us who some would call overachievers or Type A personalities will understand the idea that there is a lot of saving grace in planning for the worst and hoping for the best. A well-ordered life was quickly turned into chaos and so Tim and Darcy did what they did best... they made a companion to the "Bucket List" – a "Honey Do List"; and in this case it was a tandem effort. The living in-between time became filled with concrete tasks so that Tim could leave his family a legacy of his love that would transcend time and space.

"Father's Day 2010 was an event that Darcy planned with great care in order to surprise and surround Tim with his four children and grandchild; their happy faces were broadcast to all of us on the CaringBridge. That picture did speak a thousand words; words of togetherness and happiness and living into the moment at hand.

"At the beginning of August Tim experienced a downward spiral and it became clear that the cancer was taking greater hold of his body. Tim's choice was to continue with chemotherapy or accept that his time living in-between was going to have greater quality if he were to move to comfort care. During a church meeting where the leaders share their joys and concerns, an elder asked the question, 'So how is Tim doing with this?'... this being the knowledge that his time with us was going to be in shorter supply than when he was first diagnosed. It was easier to answer the question because of the gradual transformation that had unfolded over the summer. Tim had written in an earlier journal entry that he was prideful and stoic and yet throughout the summer there was visible evidence of a man changed by his timeline. He had become humble enough to let people he didn't even know help him; he allowed his sons the opportunity to be the "men of the house" and became openly affectionate towards Frankie. He and Darcy became closer than ever during their ten years of marriage. Tim's faith in God grew stronger as his sharper edges began to soften.

"And then of course, there was the steroid phase... or shall we call it the "Super Coop" phase when Tim could be found mowing the lawn, vacuuming the pool, walking Taffy and watching sports with Frankie — all at the same time — no, I am so not kidding! The steroids bought him more quality time for when Emily and Parker visited in late summer. Steroids gave him the energy to put Frankie on the bus for the first day of school.

"He and Darcy began to plan for this very day (the funeral) and talk about his wishes for when he was gone from her. It was a poignant and tender time when only a strong and abiding trust in life everlasting carried them through. The workaholic Tim continued to work, only this time for different reasons. He was going to work as long as he could in order to continue to provide for his family. But the cost to his health did not matter to him as much as the knowledge that his untimely death could not be a further financial burden.

"Those of us present on September 19th in this space (the church) will remember that Darcy preached about church family and God's parental love for us all. We prayed for Tim with certainty and hope that going home to be with God was a wondrous gift for all of humankind.

"The date of the benefit was changed from what was ironically yesterday's date to a time just before Tim's health began to decline again. Everyone present likely can still remember and marvel at the spirit of laughter and joy that was tinged with sadness at the fire hall that night.

"Last weekend when Tim was admitted to Hospice it truly became a plan for living — living into the last of his time in-between. He lived all week as a man of strength and surprises. At times he even seemed to mimic Lazarus. There was time enough for those who did not have the luxury of time with Tim prior to his illness. There was space for family and friends to bid farewell. One of Tim's last suppers was communion and he managed to shift the mood in the room by asking for a "chaser." It was life in full circle for Colin and Matthew (Tim's sons) to be the ones to tuck Dad in. There was time for one last phone call to daughter Emily, who carries Tim's second grandchild which continues the circle of life. It was a sweet moment of kisses all over Frankie's face from Tim, who will likely remember the second biggest Sabres fan every time he laces his skates and hits the ice to play hockey. Finally, there was time for one last silly remark from the amazing and courageous woman who can rest assured that she left no stone unturned to ensure her husband's care and comfort was continuous and loving as long as he was living.

"None of us know how much in-between time we have; however we can learn from Tim that it is not how much time we have but how well we live into that time that creates the legacy of love we leave."

Wow, that was a pretty amazing summary of the last five months of Tim's life. Thank you, my dear friend! I do remember that last Sunday Tim was in Hospice. Frankie had come to visit and when he was leaving, Tim plastered his face over and over again with kisses. Frankie, being an eight year old boy, definitely is NOT a fan of kisses. But he tolerated it well, and perhaps even welcomed it. I think in his young mind, somewhere he understood the significance. It was the last time Tim would see his youngest child.

Next, my niece Gina did another New Testament reading. "A reading from Second Corinthians. For which cause we faint not; but though our outward man perish, yet the inward man is renewed day by day. For our light affliction, which is but for a moment, worketh for us a far more exceeding and eternal weight of glory; While we look not at the things which are seen, but at the things which are not seen: for the things which are seen are temporal; but the things which are not seen are eternal. For we know that if our earthly house of this tabernacle were dissolved, we have a building of God, a house not made with hands, eternal in the heavens." The theme of these verses is consistent and completely in sync with what our lives were and beliefs became.

My minister then gave the homily. "You've already heard at least two really good sermons this afternoon, so I'm not going to try to compete with those. But I do want to share with you just a brief reflection on that one reading from Romans. I wouldn't say it was my insistence, but I encouraged Darcy to think about this passage. This is a slightly different version than was read earlier. 'Likewise, the Spirit helps us in our weakness. For we do not know how to pray as we ought, but that very Spirit intercedes with sighs too deep for words. And God who searches the heart, knows what is the mind of the Spirit because the Spirit intercedes for the saints according to the will of God.'

"I was with Tim and Darcy on Thursday and at that point Tim had become unresponsive. He was sleeping. His sleep was interrupted only by a deep sighing about every 15 or 20 minutes. And he would be laying there very peaceful and then all of a sudden he would go 'Aaaaah.' After spending perhaps an hour there talking with Darcy, we prayed together for Tim and with Tim there around the bed. I said to Darcy 'You know Darcy, I just can't get that passage out of my head from Romans where it talks about the Spirit interceding for us with sighs, too deep for words.' I have no doubt that it was the Spirit of God interceding for Tim at that very moment, ushering him from this life into that life to come.

"You know, part of this, well, a huge part of this feels so wrong, which is the fact that a wonderful, gifted father and grandfather and husband and friend died too young. But I was also struck at the funeral home last night by the boards and the pictures and even in the casket itself! I hope all of you got to see that. Tim had a kind of parting shot. 'Please put a crossword puzzle and pencil in the casket,' and Darcy put in a flashlight just in case he woke up. (Reverend Miller was chuckling at this point.) Tim was a man of humor, of great humor. Of great dry wit. And it never seemed to escape him. Not even last Sunday when I was there serving communion and he indeed took the juice and said 'chaser!'

"Tim loved life. And I think he loved life more since May, than maybe he was able to love life in all the years prior to that. And maybe that indeed is the lesson for us. Maybe that's the thing Tim has to teach us. To not wait for a diagnosis. To not wait until the end is clear, but to grab a hold of life, a hold of those we love, to let them know it, to live each and every day fully. I think Tim was able to do it and do it with such confidence because of his faith. Not a faith that he trumpeted. Not a faith that he even necessarily pursued, but a faith that he came to because of his commitment to Darcy and Frankie. He sat many Sundays in this sanctuary, right over there. I think he absorbed that Spirit. It became a part of him. It upheld him and it sustained him. Thanks be to God for the life and witness of Timothy M. Colvin. Amen."

Then our associate pastor prayed, and led us in the Lord's Prayer. After that, there was a commending of the body and spirit. We had gotten much closer to Reverend Taylor over the summer. Reverend Miller was on sabbatical from June 1st until October 1st so Reverend Taylor was the one who would occasionally come over and talk with us and pray with us. I felt truly blessed to be able to have both of them officiate at the service.

Next, Tristan sang a song I had picked out. Tristan played with me in our contemporary worship group at church. He had been there long before me, I think. And he was our one actual professional in the band who has recorded music. An excellent musician whose voice I love. I was thrilled when he agreed to sing "Save a Place For Me," by Matthew West. It's a beautiful song that addresses a loved one who has recently died. It talks about being reunited in heaven one day. The words, coupled with Tristan's beautiful, haunting voice, undid any composure I had left at this point. I melted like butter in my pew, upheld only by the strength of my sisters.

Last was the Benediction, chosen from the Roswell book of prayers, given by Reverend Miller. "God's purpose stands firm, and you His little one, need only one thing. Trust that God is able and willing to satisfy your needs. This is the essence of it all. God is love. God loves you. God carries your burdens. Amen."

The same song "Everything is Grace" was played when we left the sanctuary with the casket.

We then walked down the street to the cemetery. When I say we, I mean Reverend Miller and I. He took my hand and walked me there, keeping me steady. There was a story even behind that. It was a lovely day out and Tim liked the thought of us going to see him after church on Sundays. However, there was a little snag with the funeral home people. It was run by a man and his son. I had told the son at the church that I wanted to walk to the cemetery after the service and he told me I had to ride in the limo, even though it was just down the street. He then sent his father over who put a condescending arm around my shoulder and told me "We are just going to do this like we always do or you will screw up all the cars." Well, I knew better than to accept that. So I just fetched good 'ol Summer. I let her know what happened and she took care of things in no time flat. No one messes with Summer. She made short work of those boys.

As Reverend Miller and I stood there, waiting for everyone else to arrive, I was shocked that Tim and I had left this little detail out. No thoughts whatsoever as to what to do at the cemetery. Reverend Miller chuckled and said he could handle it, and of course he did. Then back to the church for a luncheon, which I remember very little of. I do know we had tons and tons of food left over.

• **Monday, October 18, 2010 8:04 AM**
Guestbook entry from Mom B
Darcy and Frankie, You both were in my thoughts all weekend. I wish I could have been there to offer an additional shoulder to lean on. This journey you have been on has been long and you will continue to face others as you go forth. Let family, friends and faith help you through this transition. I do not believe that time heals; it only makes what has happened easier to accept and continue with a somewhat normal existence. The sense of loss is always there.

Memories of Tim and the wonderful years you shared together will brighten up your days and your nights. Love, Mom B.

Ah, the nights. I dread those the most.

Chapter Eighteen:
On Moving Forward

• **Monday, October 18, 2010 11:54 AM**
Guestbook entry from my client
Dear Darcy, Even though I met Tim only one time, it is quite apparent how loved, admired and appreciated he was. He will be sadly missed by all that knew him. My prayers remain with you and your family. May you and Frankie find comfort in friends and family now. I hope you can all lean on each other to heal and to remember what a beautiful man Tim was and all the wonderful contributions he made in this world.

• **Friday, October 22, 2010 8:36 PM, EDT**

Surprised to hear from me? I wasn't sure if I would write again. And I'm not sure if I'll write again after this... I'm not sure about anything anymore, but they all say this is normal...

It has certainly hit me that our journey is far from over. It has significantly changed and taken a deep, deep turn in the road, but it is still a journey.

I know many of you struggle and I certainly am as well. So let's continue to use this amazing tool (CaringBridge) available to us. Feel free to sign the guestbook and write your thoughts. If you want to talk about how you are processing this — the good, bad and the ugly, please do. Some have even asked about writing Tim... Write away!

So in this way the journey hasn't changed at all. I am learning how to tolerate opposing feelings, just like accepting the diagnosis and prognosis alongside feeling gifts pouring out on us... I still feel loved and supported and blessed beyond belief, while at the same time saying that every tiny inch of this SUCKS, it all sucks...

So I don't need advice; just join me in the journey if you want to.

Okay, that was an impulsive statement to make. I need lots of advice and always do. I think maybe I meant that for people who feel like they need to say something. The truth is, they don't need to say anything. I just need people to walk beside me.

It is hard to know how to conclude a book like this, because the journey truly never ends. I am finding that writing is helpful in processing the day to day events that unfold. This book has focused on how to look death in the face, how to help someone die with dignity. I suspect then there will be a sequel to see how loss and grief takes shape in our lives in those first years after Tim's death. I am sure there will be courage required again to look at the aftermath full in the face. Somehow, I am worried that the gifts might be harder to find now with Tim gone.

There are more journal entries to come as this site was kept open for another year after Tim passed away. By the time we closed it, there were well over 15,000 hits!

I have decided to end with an excerpt I wrote for the bulletin at Tim's funeral. I don't even remember writing it, but I think it was appropriate then and it is here as well.

"While cancer is a cruel and clever disease that wreaks havoc in your life, my husband and I were able to find and experience so many gifts, treasures and healings in our lives. Since his diagnosis, we have truly been transformed, as individuals and as loving, lifelong partners. Our spiritual lives blossomed and grew in ways I would not have thought possible. And so much of that happened because of the loving, compassionate, strong hands, arms, and feet of the people of God. No one would deny that we are truly the luckiest people on earth, even with the loss we suffer. Few others could boast the kind of dedication and support we have felt poured out upon us. May God bless you one hundred fold for all the blessings you have given us. Darcy Thiel"